THE SIRTFOOD
DIET

Guide to lose weight, burn fat and being healthy, activating your skinny gene. Includes weekly meal plans, recipes for beginners and intermittent fasting lifestyle

ADELE ADANI

TABLE OF CONTENT

INTRODUCTION

Losing weight quickly, is the goal of many people. However, big mistakes are often made that can endanger health. Unfortunately, like all dreams, this also can be an unrealizable one.

Not everyone, in fact, can lose excess pounds quickly, at least not in a correct way and without damaging health. The paradox is to risk getting back the pounds lost as soon as you finish dieting.

Even if experts recommend slow but constant weight loss, it is still possible to lose weight quite quickly, following easy to read but sometimes difficult to put in action measures.

Among these we can remind you about having a healthy and balanced diet, drinking at least 2 liters of water and above all doing sport exercises to activate the metabolism and reinforce the mind. Help can also come from physiotherapy and alternative medicine, avoiding, however, very common mistakes such as DIY diet, medications and fasting. And last but not least we want you to explore the last discovery made by the two nutritionists Aidan Goggins and Glen Matten.

It's called Sirtdiet, "the lean gene diet". This innovative diet is based on two phases: first slimming and after maintenance, using the so-called Sirt foods. They activate sirtuins, a group of genes that stimulate the metabolism and burn fat. In other words, Sirt foods are capable of activating the same genes of thinness stimulated by fasting.

When it comes to diets, we are all very skeptical. A bit like the seasons, or fashions, diets come and go. If you manage to lose weight in the short term, in the long term you will be back to where you started. Of the hundreds of millions of people who follow popular diets, less than 1% will normally lose weight permanently. There is clearly a problem.

However, the diet developed by the two renowned nutritionists in the United Kingdom and Ireland, is based not only on the calorie restriction but also on eating the Sirt foods.

Only by combining these two points it is possible to lose weight. Taking Sirt foods will allow you to lose weight and not get back the lost pounds. Adopting these eating habits will achieve the well-being of your body.

The Sirt diet is a dietary regime with the characteristic of not excluding any food, but of promoting the consumption of certain foods of vegetable origin mostly. These foods contain polyphenols that stimulate the production of some proteins, sirtuins, capable of promoting weight loss and maintaining muscle mass.

Sirtuins are present in the human body and are able to optimize various functions, from the metabolic one to everything needed to protect our body from inflammatory processes. It is scientifically proven that some plant elements would be able to increase the levels of sirtuins in the body. Among the foods that contain sirtuins, it is certainly possible to mention red wine, cabbage, but also strawberries, onions, soy and parsley. The Sirt diet also focuses on other foods. In this category it is possible to include 85% dark chocolate, turmeric, matcha green tea, red chicory. Just like matcha green tea and most of the foods listed above, it is rich in polyphenols, plant compounds that would be able to activate sirtuins, enzymes that simulate the effects of calorie restriction and physical activity.

The Sirt diet plan consists of two phases lasting three weeks in total, following which it is possible to start including meat-based foods on your menus. Among the main guidelines to follow are calorie reduction, but also the intake of a juice made from cabbage, arugula, green apple, parsley, celery stalks, green apple, to be prepared at home. When it comes to these foods, it is undoubtedly necessary to remember that, in principle, they are valuable health allies by virtue of their content of antioxidants and anti-inflammatory plant compounds.

We conclude by recalling that, although the Sirt diet is characterized by the presence of a large number of healthy foods, the calorie restriction that it recommends can prove difficult to sustain. In light of this, if you intend to undertake it, it is advisable to consult your doctor and be followed step by step.

Let's start now to understand in detail what the Sirt Diet is.

1. LOSE WEIGHT QUICKLY

Going on a Diet

Following a slimming diet may not be rewarding and it is important to have at least one reason to remember to stay motivated. Obviously each of us must have their strengths, to refuse temptations and the desire to give up in critical moments.

The tips for a good diet start from looking for a strong motivation. Dieting is first and foremost a commitment to yourself. The first person you have to deal with is not the dietician, the partner, the parent, the general practitioner, but it is yourself. Those who really need to lose weight are aware that the path to be taken will be long, emotionally tiring.

The reasons for undertaking a diet are not only aesthetic, but also for self-esteem and, even more so, to protect health. Extra pounds are synonymous with cardiac fatigue, high cholesterol, diabetes risk, obesity, impaired blood test values and consequently a shorter life span. Regaining physical fitness means regaining well-being in order to learn a new lifestyle.

Having a goal to reach allows you to be more motivated. It does not matter which, because the fundamental thing is to identify the key to start the mechanism of weight loss. The desired results are more easily achieved only if you have a truly felt goal. In addition, patience, determination, and a good balance must be provided. Eliminating certain foods and practicing physical activity constantly, at least for half an hour a day, is an advice not to be overlooked.

The diet must represent a positive change in life and with a few sacrifices as possible, under penalty of failure. If we focus only on the physical aspect, we will probably not be able to implement a change that guarantees a rewarding result to achieve a profound inner change and psychophysical balance.

If the diet you start is finely personalized, it includes healthy food, good for the palate and also beautiful to see enough to gratify the taste and the senses, it will keep high the levels of serotonin which is the neurotransmitter of contentment. All this represents a valid antidote to resist temptations if you live with other people who eat without healthy rules.

A quick tip, before going on: if the diet is not balanced or excessively privative, to resist the temptation, which is still a source of stress that increases the cortisol hormone also responsible for weight gain, it is advisable to eat vegetables such as fennel and celery together with some almonds, instead of sugary snacks.

Strategies to Follow

It is essential to prefer quality foods, rich in antioxidants and vitamins, which have a beneficial effect on health, even if with a considerable caloric intake. The extra virgin olive oil, rich in calories, contains polyphenols essential for our health, therefore it will be an indispensable food for our diet. From the pantry it is good to eliminate junk food, that is snacks, chips, snacks, sauces rich in sugars, packaged foods, candies, sugary drinks, all substances harmful to health, and supply it with fruit, vegetables, lean proteins, whole grains and typically Sirt foods.

It should be borne in mind that a diet that produces effects on one person may not have any effect on another. For example, a bilious type will need to take carbohydrates in different quantities than the brain type. Just as a person who is thin in the upper part and fat in the lower part, needs a diet that takes into account this constitution and the different hormonal structure.

A good diet, therefore, is based on physical, psychic characteristics, habits, hormonal structure, stress and the ability to manage it. Many people gain weight under stress and there are others who lose it. Taking the wrong diet, therefore, can make you lose all enthusiasm and obtain the opposite effect.

Some strategies can help in the phase preceding the start of the diet and during. It is important to plan meals by cooking several times, keep a diary on which to note the changes, feelings, difficulties and results achieved as well as the objectives that gradually arise.

An ample strategy for completing a weight loss diet cannot do without physical activity. Increasing caloric expenditure both during movement and at rest during the period of muscle recovery promotes not only weight loss but also the production of endorphins, a hormone that makes fatigue less perceived. Physical activity also produces the irisin hormone that triggers the browning process to increase calorie expenditure and that is the conversion of white fat cells, fat deposits, into brown fat cells, optimizing weight loss. If you want to lose weight, you have to start moving again, 30 minutes of walking equals the calories of a glass of wine.

So before giving in to the do-it-yourself or the diet of a friend, it would be advisable to perform hormonal tests and have your psycho-bio-constitution assessed. It is important to use specialists.

Low Calories Diet

The etymology of the term "low-calorie diet" means controlled diet. From the Greek "dìaita" which means "lifestyle" and "hypo" diminutive particle, which means under, and caloric which means that it brings calories and energy.

The first phase of the Sirt diet will be a low calorie diet that provides a lower daily calorie-energy intake than that required by the body throughout the day. Therefore the application of the diet provides for a prescription by a qualified professional in case of need. The low-calorie diet is therefore not beneficial to healthy people in normal weight and without alteration of the metabolism.

In the last half century, there has been a proliferation of self-referential people who prescribe low-calorie diets, so rough, that they have caused a collective rejection of energy-restricted diets. Calories have become an outdated, useless, misleading and unreliable concept because everyone has their own recipe. For some dieticians, it is necessary to consume only foods that lead to metabolizing correctly. Some diets, for example, totally abolish milk and dairy products, cereals, legumes and even fresh fruit.

These attitudes constitute a real low-calorie diet, but also a diet that excludes 50% of the available foods. Obviously, by documenting the potential risks of a similar diet, it will be understood how far these strategies can result from the requirements of health and nutrition education of a balanced diet.

Paradoxically, excluding olive oil, cereals, legumes, milk, cheeses and fatty meats, and almost all the fruit, only lean meat and fish, eggs, vegetables and dried fruit would remain. In practice, a high-protein, potentially ketogenic and necessarily low-calorie diet, unless abnormal portions are used to make up for the missing calories. It is good to know that, there is no weight loss diet without the right calorie doses, otherwise you end up proposing a bogus low-calorie diet anyway.

The Sirt diet, the low-calorie diet par excellence, is inclusive, assumes a socio-sanitary function and at the same time acts as food therapy.

The variables of a diet

The diet is aimed at slimming and reducing the abdominal circumference. Overweight and even worse obesity are related to the onset of metabolic diseases which present a series of complications on the organism, worsen the quality of life, increase the risk of death and significantly increase public health expenditure.

It applies to a varied number of people, those who are overweight and those who need to normalize their health. The diet has a direct effect on physiological parameters, because it is able to reduce LDL cholesterol, triglycerides, blood sugar, blood pressure, uricemia. It serves to restore optimal physiological parameters and to improve quality and life expectancy.

The diet, in general, has its effectiveness when a trusting relationship is established between the patient and his dietician. A professional who does not have the technical-methodological knowledge sufficient to understand what the patient's goals and therapeutic priorities are, does not do a good job.

The psychological profile and behavior of the patient represent the variable that the specialist must take into account. He cannot prescribe the same diet to two different subjects, even though they share the same nutritional needs. It would be useless to provide a technically perfect low-calorie diet if the patient was not motivated or refused the proposed foods in disgust.

Obviously, the basic and essential requirements of the Sirt diet are summarized in some characteristics: food education and nutritional balance. The dietician must know how to shape the diet, guaranteeing the therapeutic objective and respecting the professional code of ethics.

The ability to interpret all these variables constitutes the difference between the various professionals and explains why not all patients get the same results with the same dietician, and why everyone prefers one diet over another.

It is not easy to make people lose weight and sometimes even reduce their cholesterol, triglycerides, blood sugar and blood pressure. However, the dietary process must be evaluated keeping in mind the general picture of the patient. Psychological stress, the preservation of social habits, the possible recurrence of the pathology, the fatigue of the organs, the onset of symptoms or discomforts of various kinds are variants that must be paid attention to, if you want to obtain the expected results from the diet.

The originality of Sirtdiet lies in the fact that foods rich in polyphenols are simply consumed. These have antioxidant properties, and presumably in turn activate sirtuins. In fact, among the foods that have made this diet worthy of note are wine and dark chocolate, which already have a place in our diet, also because their high levels of antioxidants can protect us from some chronic diseases and some tumors.

2. SIRTUIN PROTEIN

A Family of Sirtuins

Sirtuins or Sir2 proteins constitute a class of proteins with enzymatic activity. The name derives from a silencing-regulating yeast gene, implicated in the regulation of cellular development. The research on sirtuins began in 1991 with prof. Leonard Guarente. Mammals possess seven sirtuins, which occupy several subcellular compartments.

Sirtuins are classified according to their amino acid sequence. Prokaryotes are in U class. The first sirtuin was found in yeast and was called Sir2. In more complex mammals, there are seven known enzymes that act on cell regulation. These genes are referred to as belonging to different classes, depending on their amino acid sequence structure.

Our cells build seven different sirtuins that perform a variety of functions. In technical chemical language they are called SIRT1 - SIRT7. Some of them perform the normal function of regulating gene transcription. Others connect to proteins in the cytoplasm and mitochondria. Those are involved in regulating an extensive variety of processes from metabolism to neuro-degeneration. Some other proteins are specialized in removing acetyl groups, while others remove different groups such as lipids or make other modifications. Intensive study of sirtuins has revealed that in many organisms they are related to aging.

The Structure of Sirtuins

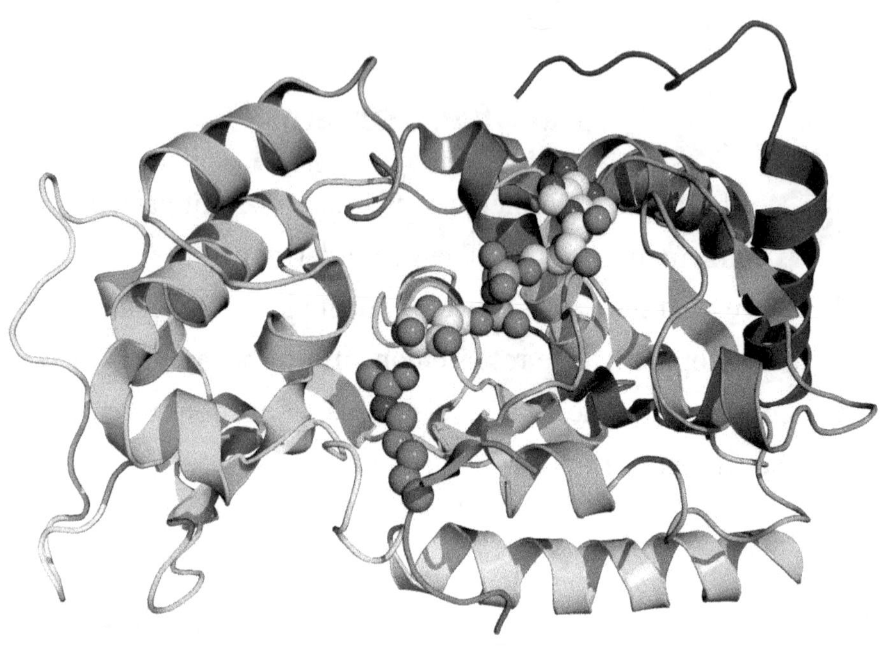

Sirtuins use a very common co-factor, NAD, to achieve an unusual reaction. They take NAD, a co-factor used in oxidation-reduction reactions, and remove its characteristic nicotinamide ring. They then extract the acetyl group from an acetylated lysine of the target protein and transfer it to the remaining fragment of the NAD molecule. All sirtuins, like Sir2 shown above, have a common structural feature. They have two domains, one can bind the NAD and takes away the nicotinamide ring, the other places the acetylated lysine near the NAD and catalyzes the transfer of the acetyl group

Physiological Role

The activity of sirtuins is inhibited by nicotinamide. For this reason it is hypothesized that the drugs that interfere with this specific receptor could increase the natural biological activities of sirtuins. The development of new agents that specifically block the nicotinamide could provide a therapeutic strategy for the development of new agents for the treatment of degenerative diseases such as cancer, Alzheimer's, diabetes, atherosclerosis, and gout. Sirtuins, in general, are part of a class of proteins that perform enzymatic activity and have the function of regulating important metabolic pathways within the body. Sirtuins are capable of regulating the physiological processes of weight loss, working on the mechanism that is put in place every time we ingest sweets or refined foods.

The mechanism of insulin that rises every time we ingest a sweet food or a refined food is the process that creates the greatest inflammation in our body. Raising insulin induces a resistance mechanism that over time creates inflammation in the tissues. An inflamed and therefore acidified tissue is the basis of every disease, especially cancer and degenerative ones. Sirtuins regulate the metabolic processes linked to insulin resistance, have control over immunity, have a fundamental role in epigenetics and are involved in defenses against tumor diseases.

Factors contributing to longevity

To explain the biological mechanisms of physiological aging and achieve greater life expectancy numerous hypotheses have been formulated and numerous studies have been conducted in different organisms, from bacteria to humans. Among the different research approaches and anti-aging interventions, the reduction in calorie intake remains the most trusted option. The restrictive regime implies one 30-40% reduction compared to the intake considered "normal" for the species in question (Ingram, Zhu et al., 2006).

Studies in numerous species (yeasts, helminths, mammals) have shown that calorie restriction (CR) can reduce the incidence and slow down the onset of age-related diseases (diseases cardiovascular and neurodegenerative), improve resistance to stress and slow down decline functional and also increase lifespan (Everitt, Roth, 2005). The effectiveness of this approach is documented by a rather full-bodied literature. The research is now aimed at establishing whether such nutritional intervention is also relevant for human aging.

The Japanese island of Okinawa has long fascinated scholars involved in anti-aging research. Between its inhabitants, there is an unusual high number of centenarians, little subject to death from diseases such as cancer and heart attack. Some rumors said that the secret of these islanders is represented by their frugal diet.

A 1978 study of Okinawans showed that the energy intake among adults was about 80% of the average Japanese. Some authors speculate that the restriction calorie may be one of the factors responsible for the longest life of the inhabitants of Okinawa (Willcox et al., 2006).

Other factors could contribute to their exceptional longevity: genetic factors, high content of antioxidants in the diet (green leafy vegetables, sweet potatoes and soy as the main protein, supplemented by low quantities of meat and fish)

Sirtuin Limits the Aging Process

According to nutritionists Aidan Goggins and Glen Matten, who have developed this diet, the consumption of certain foods would activate sirtuins, a group of genes that stimulate the metabolism, burn fat and promote fast weight loss. In addition, sirtuins are able to repair cells and improve general health by transforming themselves from slimming markers to elixirs of longevity.

The lean genes responsible for repairing and rejuvenating cells accelerate their activity by drawing on fat reserves and increasing disease resistance. The same goal can be achieved without going hungry, that is, by eating Sirt foods. Shorty fasting is a wrong attitude, because the body does not receive the necessary need for nutrients and therefore triggers a series of changes on normal growth processes to survive.

With the program of two nutritionists Aidan Goggins and Glen Matten, by introducing Sirt foods into our diet, we can lose over 3 kilos in one week, without deprivation of any kind. In addition, the "lean gene diet" proves to be an excellent tool for recovering well-being and improving the general conditions of one's health.

Effects of Sirtuins on Weight Loss

Most of the analysis of the effects of sirtuins and on weight loss were carried out only in animal laboratories, on yeasts, worms and human stem cells. Some studies have shown that an antioxidant known as resveratrol, which is found in grapes and blueberries, which activates sirtuins, can imitate the caloric restriction actions that in turn lead to weight loss. Other studies have found that resveratrol may play a role in preventing cancer, heart disease and diabetes in animals.

The addition of resveratrol in the mice diet is able to inhibit the genetic expression profiles associated with muscle aging and age-related cardiac dysfunction. However, there is insufficient evidence to understand its role in humans.

The only human evidence on the effectiveness of the Sirtfood diet, is a clinical trial, designed in a pilot study of some participants in a private gym in Chelsea, London, concerning weight loss. The Sirtfood diet was conducted over a 7 day period, 39 people lost about 3 pounds (but beyond 7 days we do not know if the calorie restriction continued, if the weight was regained or if the muscle mass was maintained).

Obviously it is a test that has many limitations. However, this pilot study is the first of many studies that should be conducted on a specific topic and should in no way be the only source of evidence to support a diet. In addition, the only participants in the study were gym goers, people who are probably health conscious and on a healthy diet regardless.

Undoubtedly genetics play a fundamental role in metabolism, which is studied by the so-called nutrigenomics, a fascinating and complex area of research. And above all still largely unexplored. The Sirtdiet clearly explains how new studies help us plan a dietary model capable of making us lose weight suffering less and aging in a healthy way. All the opposite of the magic potions that flood the web and the media, which promise miracles. The diet ensures that lost pounds will not recover, if done as needed, when you want to drop a few extra pounds or centimeters, but not for an extended period. Practicing some physical activity will certainly do well both during all its phases.

Antioxidants: Quercetin, Resveratrol, Kaempferol, Polyphenols

Antioxidants are substances capable of neutralizing free radicals and protecting the body from their negative action.

During the numerous metabolic processes, a small amount of oxygen gives rise to chemically very reactive molecules. These molecules, called free radicals, are able to damage cell structures such as the plasma membrane and DNA. The negative action of free radicals affects the health of the whole organism and accelerates the processes of cellular aging. The immune system weakens and promotes the onset of numerous diseases and tumor forms

Our organism manages to keep under control the activity of free radicals through special endogenous antioxidant substances, autonomously synthesized, and exogenous, present in food.

Quercetin is an exogenous antioxidant substance present in a large variety of fruits such as apples, grapes, olives, citrus fruits, berries, in vegetables such as tomatoes, onions, broccoli, capers and in drinks such as tea and red wine and herbal extracts. In nature, quercetin is not present in the isolated form but as an aglycone of various glycosides, including rutin and quercitrin. In this form it abounds, in particular, in the extracts of horse chestnut, ginkgo Biloba, calendula, hawthorn, chamomile, lovage and hypericum.

Resveratrol is another substance produced by different plant species which, thanks to its marked antioxidant properties, helps protect our body from cardiovascular and tumor pathologies. Resveratrol is found in berries, peanuts and pine nuts. The integration of resveratrol is absolutely impossible for commercial purposes since the individual dose required, is 3-6 grams per day.

Kaempferol, a polyphenol from endive, would be able in vitro to induce the destruction of cancer cells by apoptosis, programmed cell death and by inhibition of angiogenesis, the process that drives the vascularization of cancer cells. It is found essentially in flavonoid plants such as red onions and omega 3 fatty acids from sea bass.

Polyphenols

Polyphenols are natural organic molecules that protect cells against direct attack by carcinogens and alter their activation mechanism. Consuming regularly foods rich in polyphenols is not difficult because they abound in the vegetable kingdom and include whole grains, seasonal fruits and vegetables, suitable for a balanced diet. The best way to take advantage of the antioxidant properties of polyphenols is to eat raw or steamed foods, as cooking considerably reduces their beneficial contribution.

Polyphenols are found in many vegetables and fruits, and in other foods such as seeds and whole grains. They are more present in the aerial parts of fruit and vegetables, rather than in the stem and root, and more in the skin and in the part of the pulp closest to it and in drinks such as in red wine and tea. They are found in greater concentration in black elderberry, black currant, blueberry (Vacciniumcorymbosum), cherry and berries in general (strawberries, blackberries, raspberries), artichokes, green and black tea, filtered coffee, prunes, flax seeds, cocoa and pure dark chocolate, chestnuts, apples and 100% natural apple juice, hazelnuts, red wine, olive oil, pure pomegranate juice and soy. Spinach, black olives, broccoli, black beans, red onion and pecans also contain quite appreciable quantities of polyphenols.

The benefits of polyphenols

The benefits of polyphenols are summarized above all in the antioxidant action they perform. These substances, in fact, protect cells from damage caused by free radicals. These foods contain in large quantities these nutrients with antioxidant properties. They are able to perform different actions to bring many benefits to human health, such as the prevention of cellular aging, arteriosclerosis and cardiovascular diseases in general. Polyphenols can intervene in the early stages of cancer development, protecting cells from direct attack by carcinogenic elements. For this reason, their function is important in the prevention of certain cancers, such as that of the lung, stomach, oesophagus, pancreas, liver and skin. Their anti-inflammatory action is ensured by the fact that they are able to inhibit the intervention of arachidonic acid. They also have a non-indifferent antibacterial and antiviral action.

The Advantages of Sirt Foods

The scientific reason behind the Sirt diet lies in the fact that sirtuin activators would have several health benefits, including fat removal, building muscle, suppressing appetite, improving memory and controlling sugar, and cleansing from free radicals that accumulate in cells in the blood. Undoubtedly, several of the foods included in the diet, the sirtuin-stimulants, are rich in substances such as resveratrol and flavonoids, for which several studies have ascertained positive effects for health as we already explained. Resveratrol, for example, is a good antioxidant, anti-inflammatory and protective vessel, as indeed some flavonoids, for their part, have hepatoprotective and antioxidant actions.

Compared to many other unbalanced diets, which focus more on weight loss, the Sirt diet plans to take foods that excellently regulate the entire metabolism and burn fat, in addition to improving the health of the cells and promoting the increase of muscle mass, which turns out to be perfect for those who already train constantly in the gym. The role of sirtuins consists mainly in checking that the genes remain active or inactive in particular situations. Hence, when DNA damage occurs, they not only regulate the repair mechanism, but improve the general health of the cells. Sirtfood is a diet that is based on the inclusion and not on the exclusion of food, which allows you to lose even more than 3 kilos in a week. And if some of these foods are not so well-known, most of them are foods known and used in traditional cooking.

Fresh, genuine, easily available and suitable for our palate (strong references to the Mediterranean diet) that combined with each other or with other ingredients give rise to tasty dishes: from stir-fried prawns to scrambled spicy eggs, from pasta to smoked salmon with chocolate truffles. All so good and simple that you will even forget to be on a diet. The strong points of the diet can be summarized in some fundamental characteristics. First of all, it is balanced and healthy, with easy-to-follow recipes that are part of our daily lives. It is compatible with all food regimes and is based on inexpensive and easily available products. It does not force us to prohibit renunciations and lose weight without losing muscle mass. It does not upset habits, does not ruin social life and does not recover lost pounds, there is no sense of hunger. Finally, it helps keep cholesterol, blood sugar in check and is approved by doctors and nutritionists.

The disadvantages of Sirt foods

Weight loss, for those who follow this type of diet, is mainly due to the fact that the foods included in the menu are low in calories and fat. There are few scientific studies to support this theory. However, experts say, the link between sirtuin production and weight loss, as well as that between specific genes and weight loss, is far from certain.

Even assuming that sirtuin activates metabolism-related genes, at the moment we do not know for sure whether it also activates genes that have the opposite effect at the same time. And to fully understand the genetic action of a food, it would be necessary to carry out studies that involve the use of complex bioinformatics tools. It is a diet that involves a strong calorie restriction practiced in a very short period of time. It is a lightning diet, 3 weeks, that many other lightning diets are likely to run into the much feared "recovery effect"

This diet regulates the consumption of few carbohydrates and few proteins. In fact, there could be tiredness, fatigue, headache and pressure drops. Tolerating the daily ingestion of smoothies and vegetable concentrates for three weeks is not allowed for everyone. In fact, nausea and intestinal disturbances could be registered.

The Sirt diet is strongly discouraged for children and adolescents, people who are underweight, deteriorating or recovering, and in the presence of nutritional deficiencies or eating disorders. In addition, it should only be followed on advice and medical supervision by pregnant or breastfeeding women, elderly people and menopausal ladies, and in case of diabetes, metabolic diseases, liver and kidney problems, gastrointestinal disorders and chronic conditions.

However, it is good to keep in mind that this diet should not always be followed. For some people it will be necessary to repeat it only twice a year, for others once every three months. This depends on the metabolism and many factors that vary in each of us. Our advice is always to go to a specialist when deciding to start a new diet.

3. THE SIRT FOODS

Lose Weight by Eating

Sirt foods are foods capable of activating proteins in our body, sirtuins, which help not to accumulate fat and fight against free radicals and diseases, and also stimulate the metabolism, burn fat and promote loss. We will see what these foods are and how to bring them to the table so as not to lose their precious properties.

All the plant foods contain bioactive molecules that are good for the body. However, it is good to have a deeper knowledge in the vast variety of Sirt foods, which also includes foods that are hardly imagined to be part of a weight loss diet, such as red wine, which contains sugars and alcohol, and chocolate, which in turn is a high calorie and sugary food. Both of them have a bad reputation for healthy eating. In addition to foods such as strawberries, blueberries and citrus fruits, walnuts, buckwheat, red pepper and green tea, cabbage, radicchio, red onion and arugula are well suited to a diet. The exceptional peculiarity of this diet, which makes it almost unique, is the fact that it is based, as has been stated, on the inclusion and not on the exclusion of food.

They are all foods that are part of the sirtfood diet, born from genetic studies, based on the activation of the "lean gene" to lose weight in a healthy and fast way, preserving energy, muscle tone and a good mood.

Certain richer dihydrate foods are certainly recommended as a basket on which to base a tasty, healthy and satisfying diet. Chili peppers, dark chocolate (with 85% cocoa), green tea, lovage, coffee, nuts (maximum 3 per day), citrus fruits, blueberries, capers, soybeans are among the elements of which you can't do without in a sirtfood diet. Among the vegetables, cabbage, celery, red radicchio, red onion, rocket and parsley are indispensable. Buckwheat, dates and turmeric are considered to be "must eat" in the Sirt diet. Another important source of the sirtuin activator called fisetin is the strawberry, to be eaten in large quantities

The point is that the shelves of supermarkets are full of products prepared using refined flours, sugary drinks, sweets full of glucose syrup designed to satisfy the desire for sweet and fat that we have inherent in us.

In fact, even if we live in a constantly evolving world, our genes have not followed this same evolutionary path and have remained the same as when man hunted for food. In such difficult times, being able to get abundant and fatty food could mean more energy and more chances of survival to defend yourself from attacks or even prepare for periods of fasting and hunger.

This is the explanation of why there is still the desire to eat energy-rich foods, but this is also the main problem, because when we eat abundantly we also send a precise signal to the body. In particular, genes are activated, called the aging genes, which, on the one hand, allow cells to produce more energy with the consequent production of free radicals which are transformed in body fat.

The solution is to avoid extreme diets, fasts, or food regimes that simply aim to deprive the person of any food considered prohibitive as carbohydrates and sweets. The risk is not only to increase sadness and depression but also to follow unregulated diets that do not provide the right nutrients.

A balanced diet

The solution could be to follow a balanced diet, which favors unrefined foods, fruits and vegetables rich in fiber and antioxidants and which limits the consumption of sugar. Without neglecting foods particularly rich in substances, such as anthocyanins, resveratrol, epigallocatechin gallate, capsaicin or quercetin, capable of activating sirtuins, a group of 7 proteins perform different functions in the body, for the production of antioxidant enzymes.

Sirtuins are involved in the regulation of metabolism. They transport the fat reserves from the fat cells to the blood to then convert them into energy, and they control the inflammatory processes and the cycle of life. In fact, sirtuins are able to silence the genes of aging with the double result of accumulating less fat and having less free radicals in the body, losing weight, living longer and stay healthy. In fact, sirtuins deceive the body and send a signal that makes us believe that we are fasting, that we are entering a period of famine and that survival is at risk, when in reality it is not and we are eating.

This signal from sirtuins activates the genes responsible for survival, all resources are activated, all the available energy is used. Free radical damage is repaired to protect us from disease and fat does not accumulate. As said, you lose weight and live longer with help to fight age-related diseases.

Many "SirtfoodDiets" were launched in the United States: dieticians and nutritionists have begun to encourage the consumption of foods that activate sirtuins for weight loss, to increase energy, to reduce stress levels, but also to extend life expectancy.

To be honest, a dark chocolate and red wine diet is quite appealing. In addition, to have the positive effects of foods that activate sirtuins, it is enough to make a balanced diet of them. They are foods rich in particular nutrients that help the production of the so-called "lean gene" faster than our body would normally do. To know more accurately the most important foods that can help wake up and regulate our metabolism thanks to the Sirt diet, a list of the 20 most important foods will follow.

Red Wine

Red wine is the original Sirtfood, the one from which the research at the base of this diet started and which sparked all the frenzy born around these foods.

Red wine is an alcoholic drink typical of the Mediterranean area, obtained by fermentation of black grape must. Red wine is famous for its organoleptic properties (extremely variable according to its type) and for its nutritional characteristics. Containing ethyl alcohol, red wine cannot be considered a real "healthy" drink; on the other hand, thanks to the presence of phenolic antioxidants, it shows some health benefits. Generally, when we talk about the benefits related to the consumption of red wine, the first molecule that comes to mind is resveratrol (on which there are dozens of approved scientific studies). Its resveratrol content, along with another key sirtuin activator, piceatannol, is believed to be one of the key motivations for lifespan. It also protects the brain from cognitive decline related to Alzheimer's disease. Metabolic properties of antioxidant, antibacterial, antifungal, anti-tumor, anti-inflammatory and blood fluidization properties are attributed to this non-flavonoid phenol.

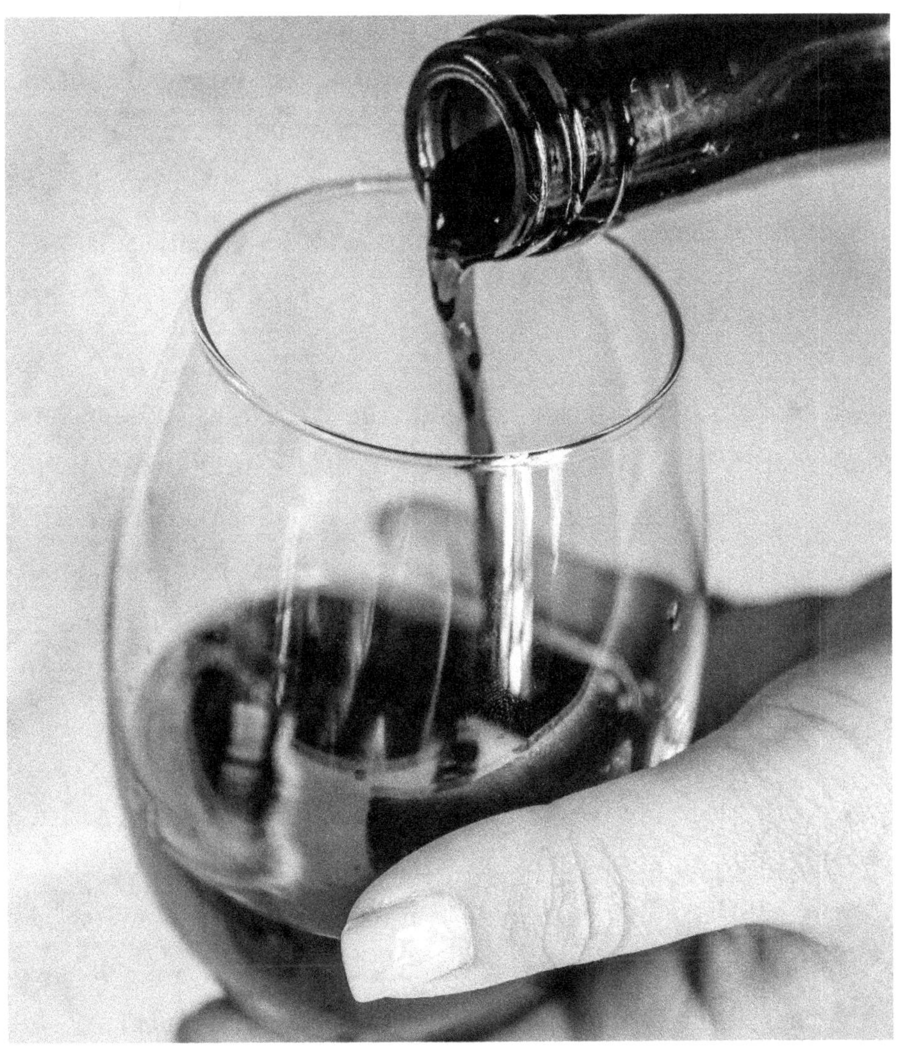

As if that were not enough, red wine is also rich in quercetin. This flavonoid (tetraoxyflavonol) represents a metabolic inhibitor of some enzymes involved in the inflammatory response. The antioxidant functions of quercetin are to restore tocopherols (vit E), detoxify cells from superoxide and decrease the secretion of nitric oxide during inflammation.

Furthermore, according to the "American CancerSociety", this flavonoid acts as a powerful anti-cancer, especially in the colon.

Red wine is rich in so-called tannins, also known as proanthocyanidins; these phenolic compounds, responsible for the red pigment, are very famous for their potential beneficial action at the cardiovascular level (similar to that of the various molecules mentioned above).

Cocoa

To be considered a true sirtfood, chocolate must be dark and contain at least 85% solid cocoa. Chocolate is often treated with alkalizing agents to reduce acidity and give it a darker color. This treatment is known as the "Dutch method" and drastically decreases the content of sirtuin activating flavonoids, compromising the healthy properties of the product. Epicatechin pigments are the activating nutrients of sirtuin.

An Aztec legend gives birth to the cocoa tree, from the sacrifice of a queen. With her husband at war, the queen was the custodian of the wealth of the kingdom. When the enemies tried to ask her where the treasures were hidden, she fell silent and was punished with death. From his blood, according to the Aztecs, this plant with exceptional fruit was born. Legends aside, the history of cocoa is truly ancient.

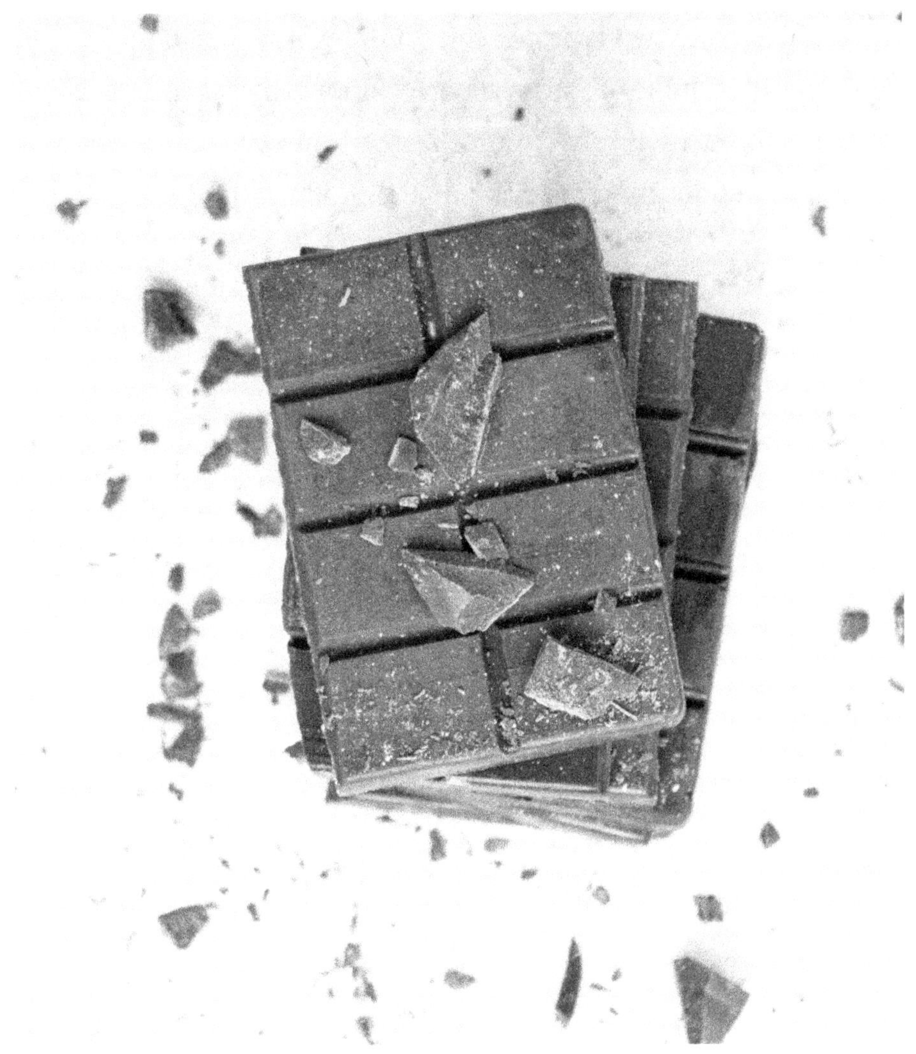

Traces of cocoa have recently been discovered on containers belonging to a community lived in Ecuador about 5300 years ago, dating back the first known use of cocoa for more than a thousand years (until now it was thought that the use of cocoa dates back to about 4000 years ago, in Mexico).

Celery

The most nutritious parts of green celery are the heart and the leaves. There are two types of celery: the white one and the green one. The bleaching of celery is a technique that was created to attenuate the particularly strong flavor of this vegetable, but also compromising its ability to activate the production of sirtuine.

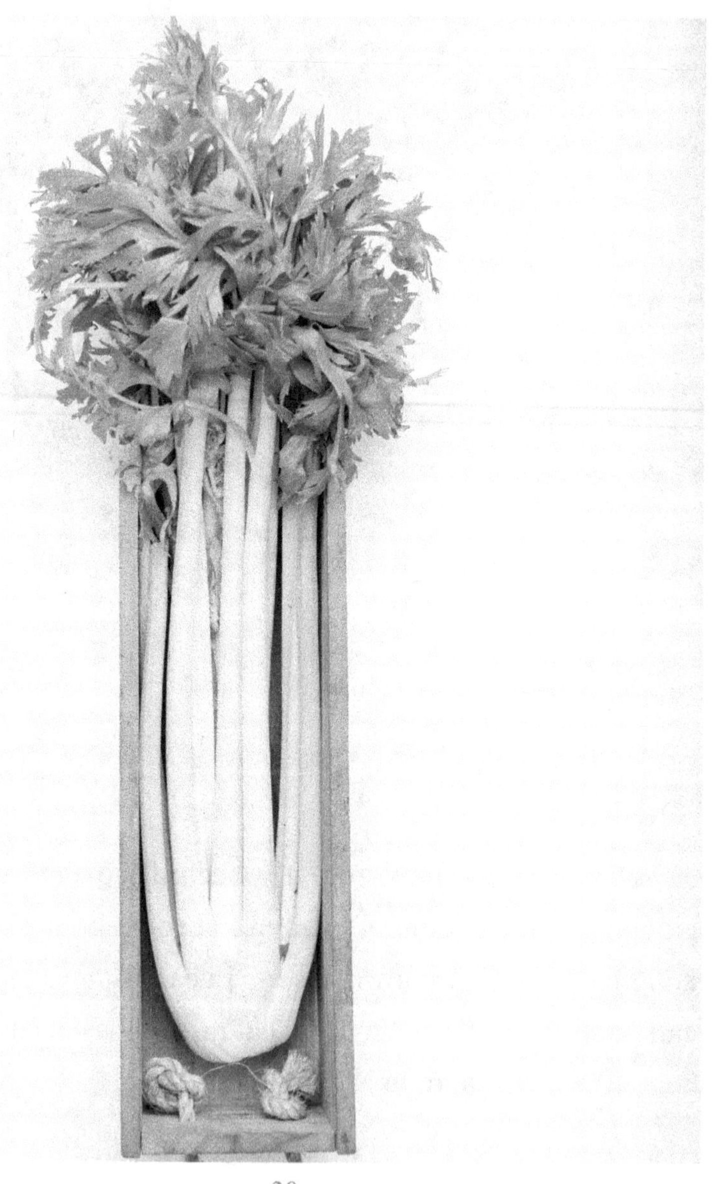

Celery boasts a very low calorie content: in 100 grams there are just 20 kcal. Water constitutes more than 88% by weight, while the remaining 12% is divided between carbohydrates, proteins, fibers and fats (very few). In addition, celery represents a source of mineral salts, such as iron, manganese and potassium, as well as being rich in antioxidants (vitamins A, C and E). Apigenin and luteolin constitute the activating nutrients of sirtuin.

Chili Pepper

Hot chilli is a fantastic sirtuin activator and a formidable metabolism activator.

Chilli is a food that falls into the VI and VII fundamental group of foods. It is a vegetable used mainly as a spice, fresh or dry. In other countries, for example in Central and South America, thanks to the habit for the spicy taste, large quantities of chili are eaten every day.

Chili peppers have a moderate energy intake, mainly provided by carbohydrates (fructose); proteins are very scarce, as are lipids.

It is cholesterol-free and contains a good percentage of dietary fiber.

Ripe chili is particularly rich in vitamins; the content in ascorbic acid is particularly relevant (229 mg of vitamin C per 100 grams of fresh fruit). Also noteworthy is the generous presence of carotenoids (precursors of vitamin A) and a moderate concentration of niacin (or vitamin PP).

The intake of mineral salts, especially potassium, is also good; the levels of calcium and phosphorus are less interesting but noteworthy.

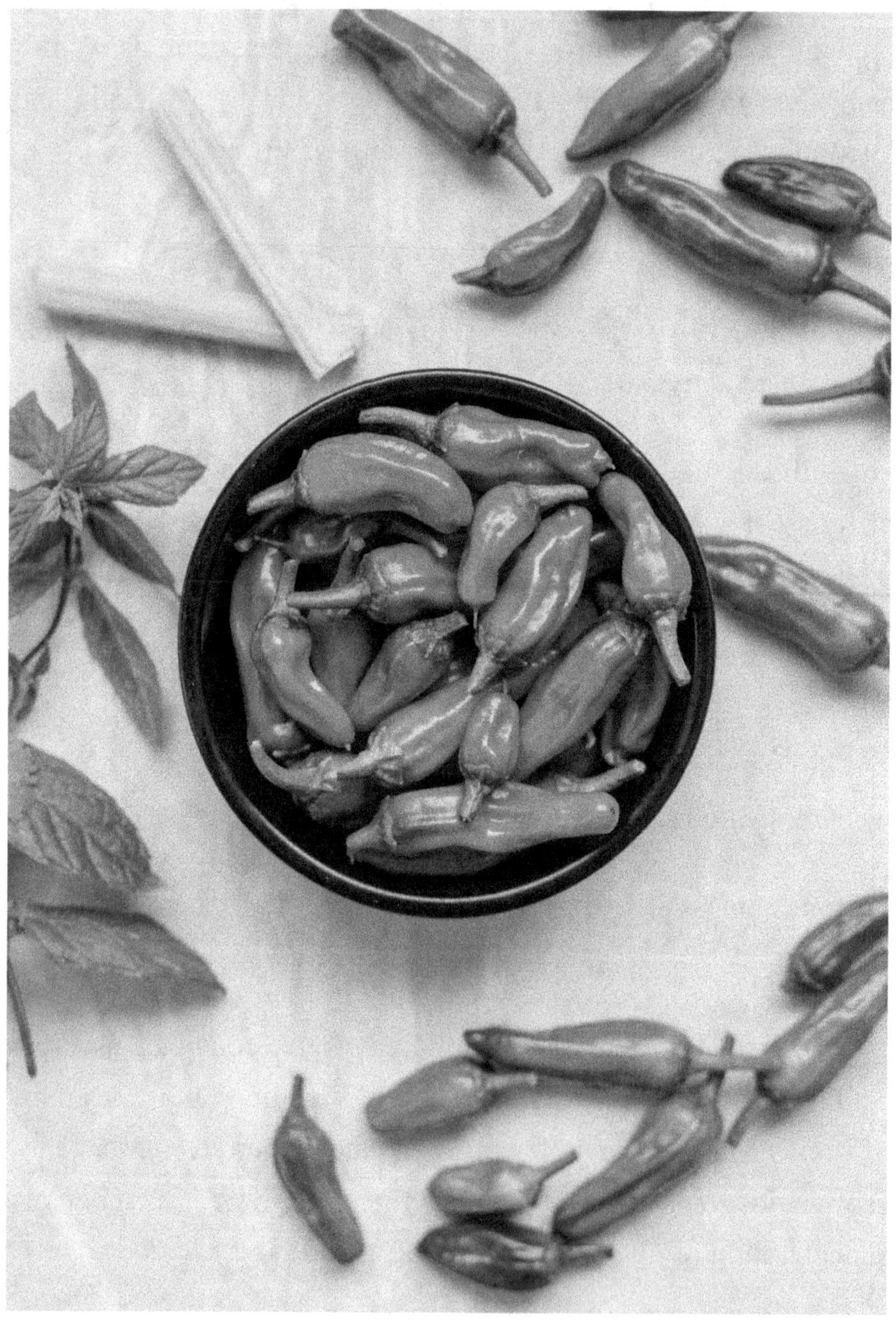

This colorful set of nutritional principles (with the exception of vitamin C), is further concentrated in the spice pepper, then in the dried and possibly powdered fruit; in the same way, the spicy flavor with which a little panache is given to the more every-day bland dishes, is also strengthened. Luteolin and myricetin are the activating nutrients of sirtuin.

Cabbage

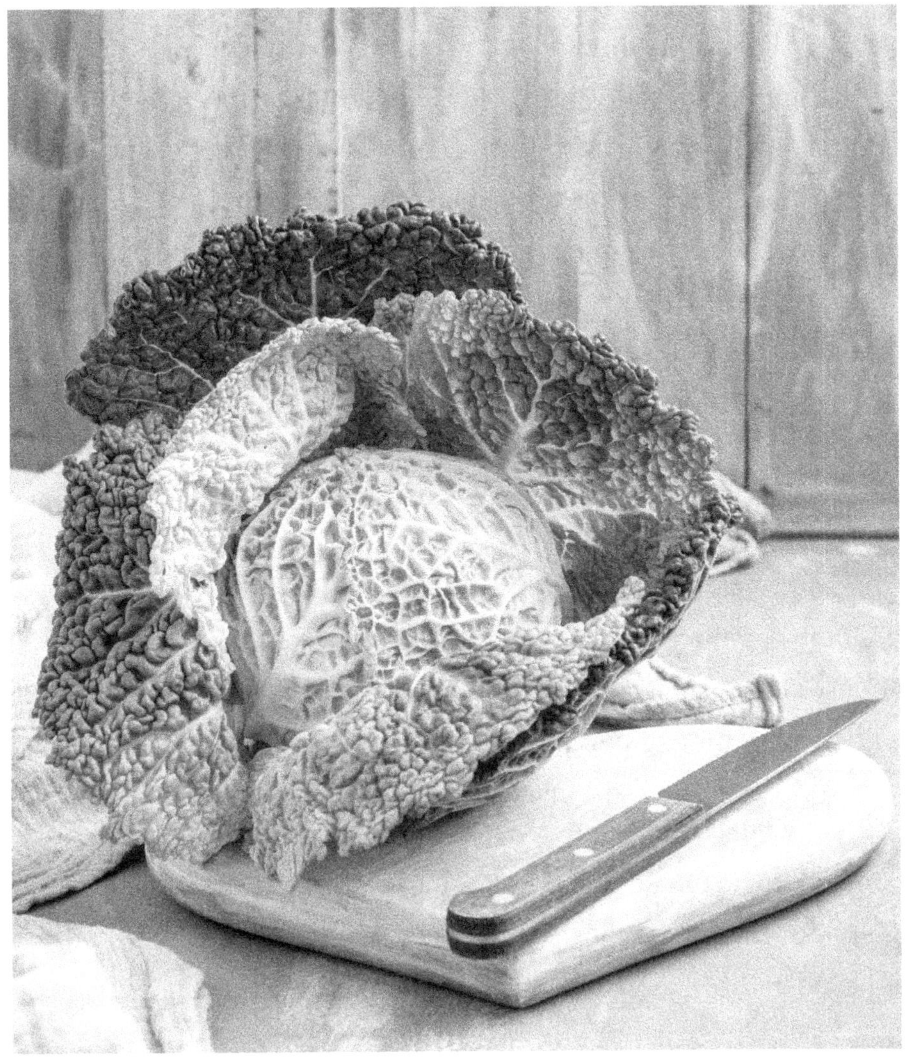

Cabbage boasts huge quantities of quercitin and kaempferol which make it a fundamental ingredient of every diet, even the Sirt one, which represent inactivating activators of sirtuin akaempferol and quercetin. It is also an autochthonous vegetable, very common and easy to find, as well as being cheap.

Cabbage and savoy cabbage are two subspecies of the well-known Brassica oleracea L. both types of cabbage (green or red) have the same botanical, chemical-nutritional (except pigment content) and cultivation characteristics and contain high quantity of vitamin C (ascorbic acid) and B-carotene (retinol eq. - pro-vitamin A); with regard to this vitamin concentration and that of many other antioxidants (especially phenolic substances), savoy cabbage and cabbage are considered protective foods against various forms of cancer. In addition, the high content of dietary fiber is definitely effective in promoting proper intestinal functioning (preventive and curative towards constipation).

Buckwheat

The proteins contained in the buckwheat seed have a good biological value. They are in fact composed both of essential amino acids, such as lysine, threonine and tryptophan, and of sulfur-containing amino acids.

Buckwheat is rich in mineral salts such as iron, phosphorus, copper, zinc, selenium and potassium. The latter even exceeds the share contained in other cereals. A valuable component, both of the seed and of the vegetable part, is represented by antioxidants.

The vitamins contained in buckwheat are mainly B1, B2, niacin (PP) and B5.

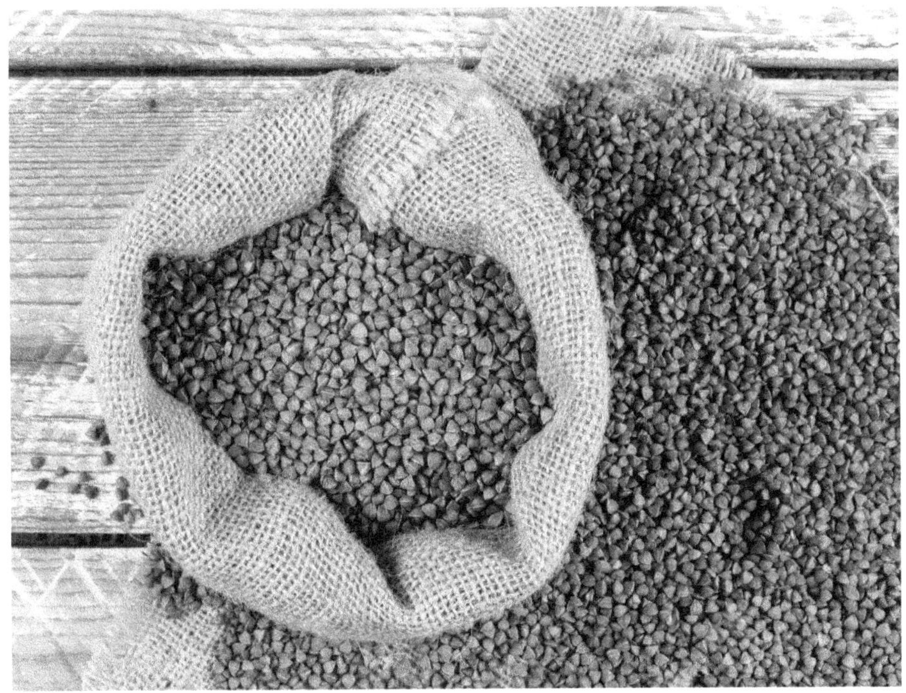

Because of its nutritional properties, and the significant food uses, buckwheat is often classified as a cereal, despite not belonging to the Graminacee family. Buckwheat possesses all the nutritional characteristics of a cereal and a legume, although it is not, from a botanical point of view, neither one (it does not belong to the Graminacee family) nor the other (it does not belong to the Legume or Fabaceae family).

Buckwheat is extremely popular in Japan and tradition has it that when Buddhist monks made long trips to the mountains, all they brought with them to make food was a pot and a bag of buckwheat. This was able to feed them for weeks.

This plant is one of the best known sources of rutin, a sirtuin activator.

Among the antioxidants present, we remember rutin and tannins, more concentrated in the herbaceous part, therefore in the leaf.

Rutin is a glycoside of quercetin, which has the strengthening value of the capillary wall as its health value. Rutin-based products can therefore prevent the appearance of bleeding, improving microcirculation and exhibiting a marked anti-inflammatory and antioxidant property. In addition to the presence of rutin, buckwheat contains other flavonoids, such as vitexin, isovitexin, orientin and quercetin.

Buckwheat, thanks to its ability to provide energy and "vigor", can be introduced in the diet for athletes, for pregnant women and for elderly people. Furthermore, as mentioned, it can also be taken by celiac people

Always remaining in the food sector, buckwheat has a defect, which is that of being a potential allergen. Food allergies to this cereal are mainly concentrated in Asia, but recently they have also appeared in Italy.

Medjool Dates

The inclusion in this list of Medjool dates can initially be very strange, considering the fact that they are 66% composed of sugar.

This substance is not connected with the production of sirtuin because it is provided with gallic acid and caffeic acid. It should be consumed in small quantities.

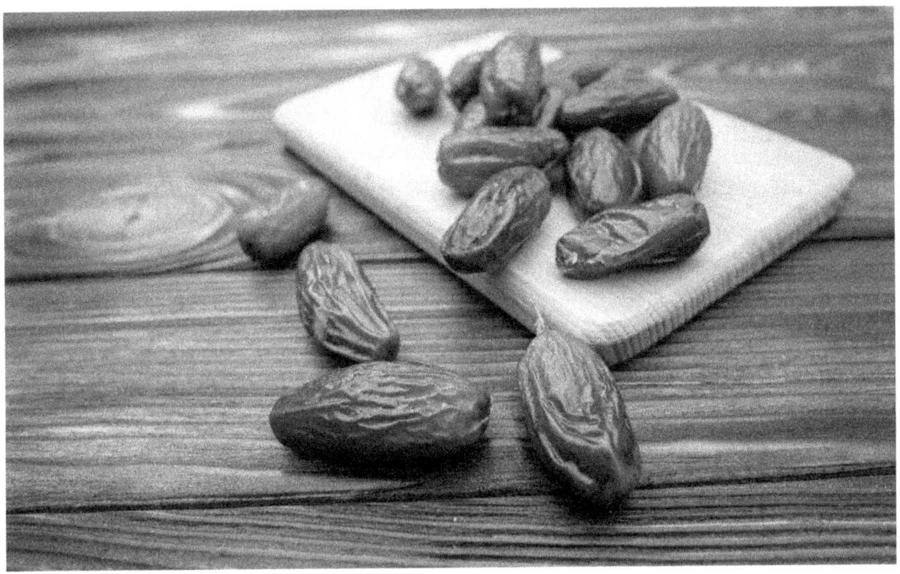

However, the sugar present in the dates is very different from the refined sugar and is balanced by polyphenols that activate the production of sirtuin.

These dates are also allies in fighting the risk of diabetes and heart disease.

It is surprising how long and productive the date palm is: some species begin to produce fruit after three years and can live for up to three centuries; under certain conditions - particularly during the full maturity of the plant (about 30 years) - date palms can produce over 50 kilos of fruit annually.

Capers

Capers are not actually fruits, but flower buds. The caper plant is widespread throughout the Mediterranean area and is rich in nutrients such as kaempferol and quercetin which favor the production of sirtuine. In the archipelago of the Aeolian Islands it has been cultivated since time immemorial, finding in this context particular vigor and exceptional vitality, thanks to the volcanic soil and the clearly favorable climatic conditions: medium wind, very low humidity.

Capers have a very low energy value, mainly provided by complex carbohydrates. Lipids are almost absent (but mainly unsaturated) and proteins (with low biological value) are not significant. There is a significant fiber content, while cholesterol is absent.

Coffee

Coffee is a real treasure trove of plant compounds with great health benefits. Coffee drinkers have a significantly lower risk of contracting certain types of cancer, neurodegenerative diseases and even diabetes. It also protects the liver and helps keep it healthy. The caffeic acid and chlorogenic acid contained in the coffee act as activating nutrients for sirtuins.

Caffeine is an alkaloid which, taken internally, exercises a discrete nerve function (which interacts on the nervous system), therefore psychotropic (which has an effect on psychic functions, specifically tends to improve the level of attention).

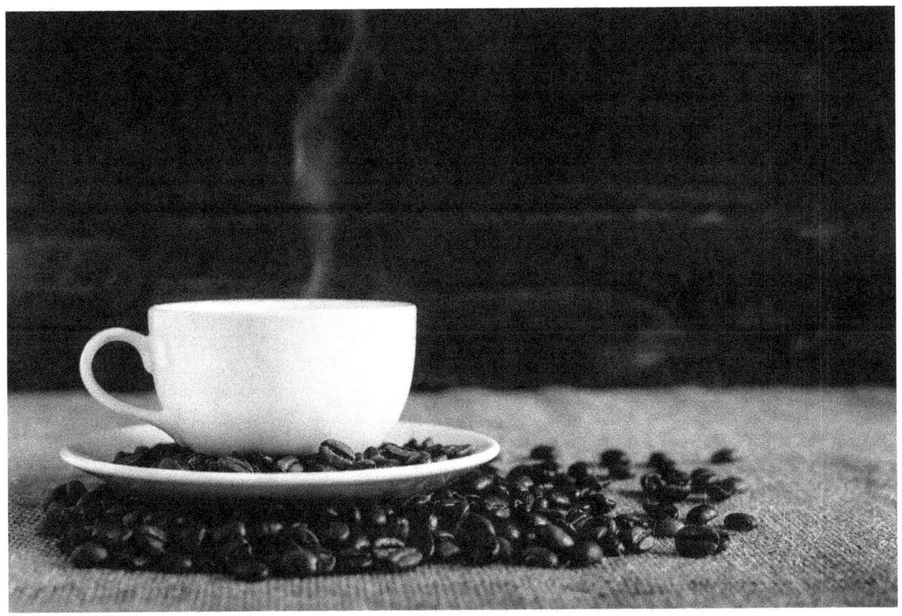

Caffeine also has a cardio-circulatory effect, acting mainly as a vasodilator and accelerating the rhythm of the heart. In addition, it appears that this methylxanthin may affect lipid metabolism, increasing the release of fatty acids by fat cells. It also has a marked diuretic function.

Caffeine, belonging to the class of alkaloids, has exciting properties on the central nervous system; in fact, it stimulates wakefulness and, because of its ability to improve muscle reactivity, it is often called "doping of the poor". It is often used for topical use for its slimming and anti-cellulite abilities;

Caffeine is contained in herbal, dietetic, cosmetic and pharmaceutical products. In particular, this methylxanthin exerts a thermogenic function, stimulating the mobilization of fats from adipose tissue and subsequent oxidation. In the pharmaceutical field, caffeine is a widely used ingredient; it is often included in the composition of important drugs such as, for example, anti-migraines.

Extra Virgin Olive Oil

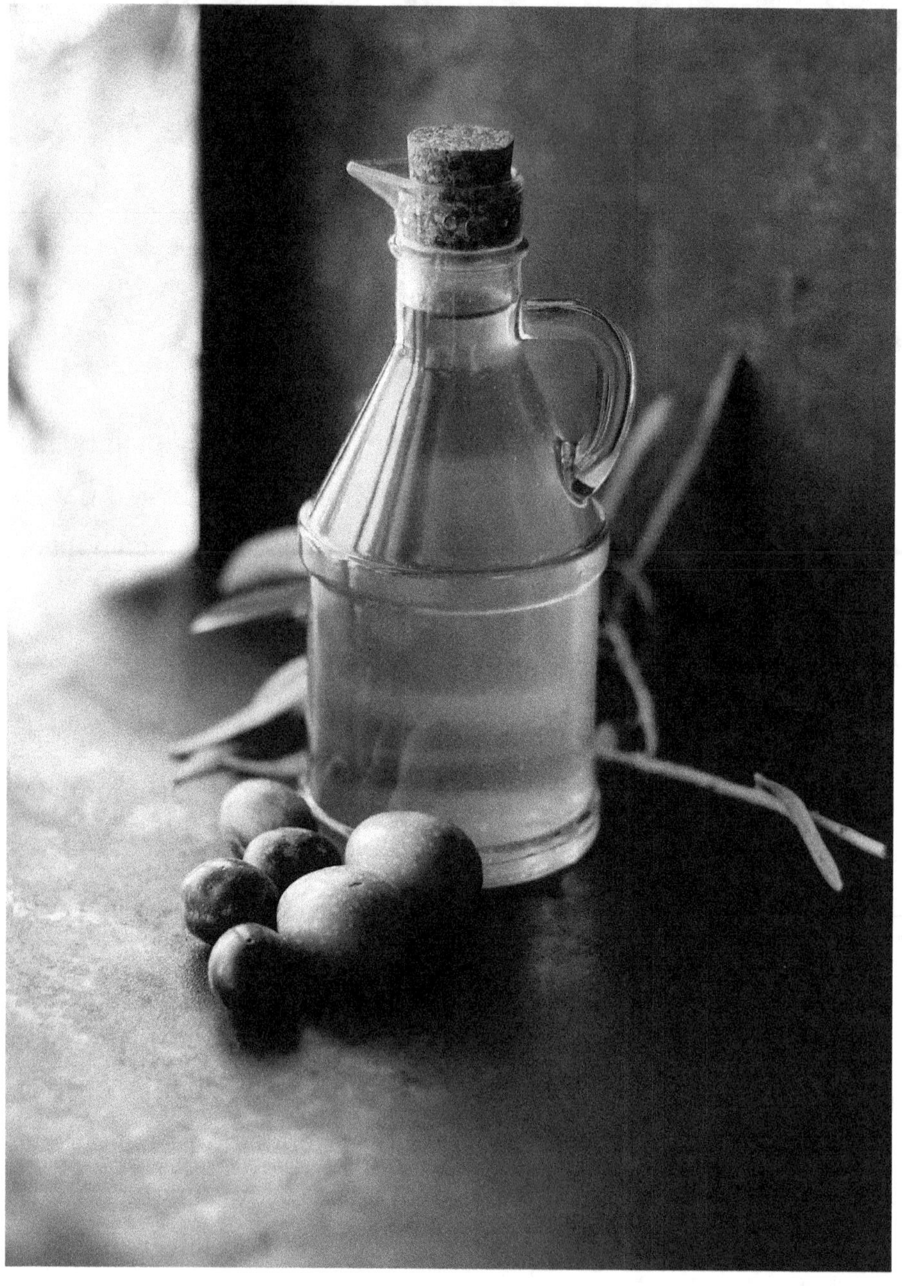

Olive oil was already mentioned by Hippocrates as "the cure of all ills", well over 2000 years before modern science proved its wonderful benefits. Oleuropein and hydroxytyrosol have the function of Nutrient activators of sirtuin

Virgin oil is obtained only through the mechanical pressing of the fruits and in conditions that do not lead to the deterioration of the oil. In this way you can be sure of the quality of the product and its polyphenol content.

Olive oil, the main food of the Mediterranean diet, is the absolute favorite condiment both raw and for cooking. Its high smoke point (210 ° C for extra virgin olive oil) makes it one of the most suitable condiments for frying. However, olive oil has a very high energy value (899 Kcal per 100 grams) and for this reason, despite its beneficial properties, it is good not to abuse it. In particular, especially in case of obesity and overweight, it is advisable to dose it with a spoon or with a teaspoon, respecting the doses provided for in the food program.

Olive oil is particularly rich in monounsaturated fats and in particular of oleic acid. Thanks to its particular composition in fatty acids, it is one of the best condiments to keep the levels of bad cholesterol (LDL) in the blood under control.

In fact, oleic acid reduces LDL-cholesterol levels without affecting the percentage of HDL-cholesterol. This fatty acid, although not essential, is therefore very important for our well-being. Oleic acid is found in numerous vegetable-based condiments and especially in olive oil which, also for this reason, represents one of the best condiments to use in the kitchen.

Matcha Green Tea

Matcha tea grows in an area exposed to shade for 90%, while the common green tea grows exposed to direct sunlight.

The matcha leaves are then chopped into a powder using a stone. Unlike green tea, which is infused and then drunk, this powder dissolves in water and is ingested.

The advantage of this method is that it allows the intake of a greater quantity of EGCG, a substance that activates sirtuin.

For some years now there has been a lot of talk about green tea products, cleverly offered to consumers as real beauty elixirs and antidotes against aging. The much-vaunted health effects of green tea are linked, for a change, to its precious content of antioxidants, which as everyone knows by now, helps the body to defend itself from free radicals (reactive molecules involved in cell damage).

In particular, the antioxidant potential of the drink is associated with the high content of catechins, which in green tea represent about 20-40% of the dry weight. Among these substances the most abundant is called (-) - epigallocatechin gallate (EGCG) and is particularly known for having demonstrated strong antioxidant and anti-mutagenic properties. Thanks to these characteristics, EGCG inhibits the growth and proliferation of cancer cells; it also reduces the levels of LDL cholesterol and triglycerides, thus exerting a protective action against cardiovascular diseases.

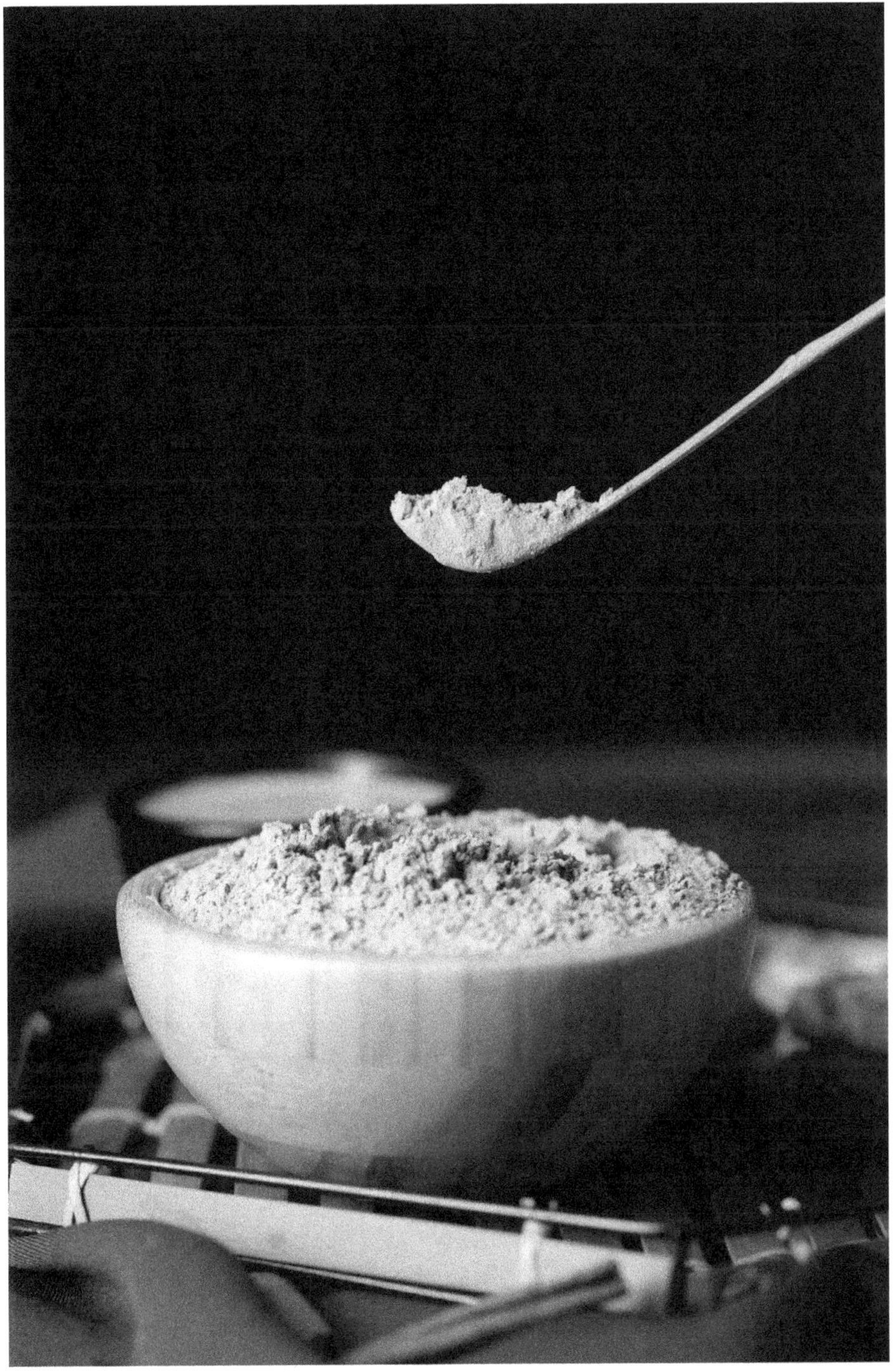

Epigallocatechin aside, the mixture of the various substances present in green tea has demonstrated an antioxidant action superior to the individual components, confirming the now accepted thesis according to which food phytocomplexes are much more active than the single isolated and purified components.

In a world where the success of a certain food or dietary supplement is increasingly linked to its real or presumed anti-aging, anti-degenerative and anti-cancer abilities, the antioxidant virtues of green tea certainly could not go unnoticed. In this regard, the Food And Drug Administration has proved cautious, due to conflicting results between the various studies. If, on the one hand, as the American body has rightly done, we must take note of the research that denies many of the alleged virtues of green tea, on the other, we cannot even ignore the increasingly numerous studies that punctually enhance them.

Lovage

Lovage is an extremely versatile plant, with a celery and parsley flavor, but much stronger. It is very rich in quercitin, a substance that activates sirtuin.

It was considered an aphrodisiac, so much so that even Charlemagne ordered it to be planted in his garden.

Unfortunately today we are no longer used to its flavor, but its beneficial properties are undeniable.

Several properties are ascribed to the lovage, including diuretic, carminative, emmenagogic, sedative and antimicrobial properties. More precisely, the naturally washing power of the urine is used to promote the resolution of infections affecting the urinary tract and to prevent the formation of any kidney stones.

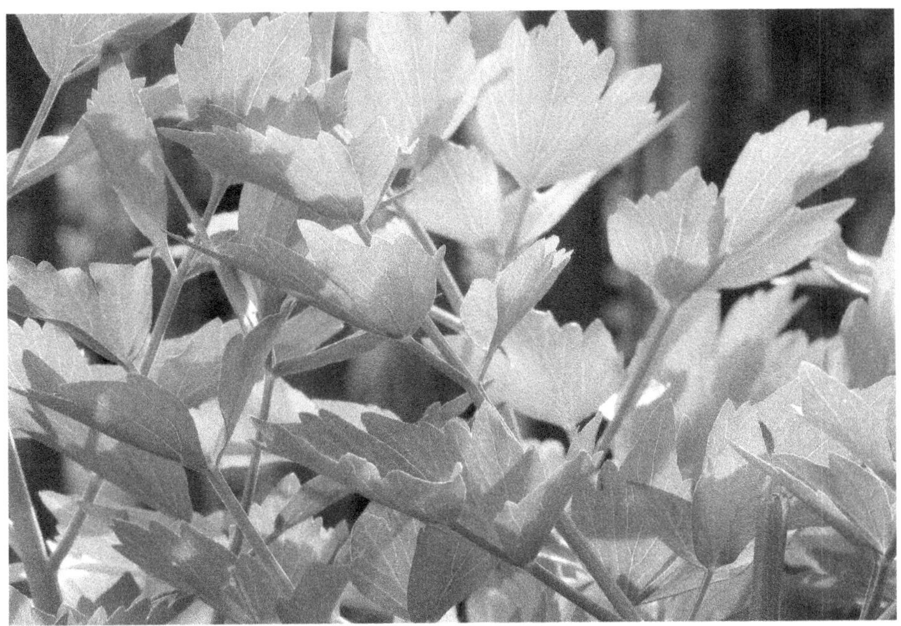

Furthermore, the lovage essential oil seems to be able to exert a spasmolytic effect on smooth muscles, thanks to the action of the ligustilide contained in it.

Finally, the plant also ascribed the ability to increase both salivary secretion and gastric secretion. This action is probably due to the alkyl phthalides contained in the essential oil and the characteristic bitter taste of the lovage.

In fact, it is not unusual for this plant to be used in digestive liqueurs or to be used for the preparation of herbal teas with indications for the treatment of dyspepsia.

Parsley

Too often in the kitchen we tend to use a small sprig of parsley for decorative purposes only.

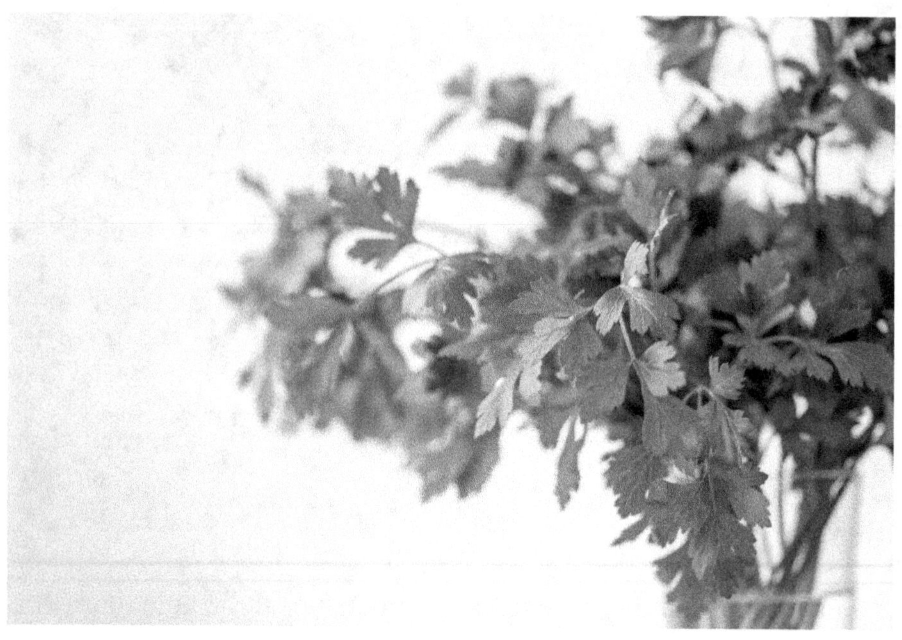

Parsley was already known at the time of Ancient Rome as a garnish to be consumed at the end of the meal to refresh the mouth.

In reality, this plant is an excellent source of apigenin, a nutrient that activates the production of sirtuin and which is rarely found in such significant quantities in other foods. Parsley (Petroselinumhortense) is a biennial plant.

It grows spontaneously in South East Europe and is widely cultivated in all temperate countries. The term parsley derives from the Greek petrosélinon, from pétra (stone) + sélinon (celery), properly celery that grows on stones.

In the kitchen, the leaves are used, mainly those that sprouted the first year, because they are more developed and valuable than those of the second. There are very few aromas that find such a wide use in the kitchen. Whether used to garnish or flavor dishes, parsley goes well with most foods, vegetables and animals.

A fresh parsley can be recognized by its bright and lively color and the pleasant aroma it gives off. It should be kept in the refrigerator and consumed within a few days. If it has sufficiently long stalks, the parsley remains green and fresh longer when it is soaked in a jar together with a cork.

Red Onion

Red onions have the highest concentration of quercitin, but yellow ones also contain significant quantities.

It is important to eat them raw, to keep the levels of nutrients unchanged: in fact fried onions lose as much as 20% of quercitin during the process, a percentage that reaches 65% if cooked in the microwave and 75% if boiled.

The strongly aromatic onion is botanically related to other spice vegetables with similar characteristics, such as garlic, leek, shallots and chives.

Inevitable ingredient of many recipes, the onion stands out for the abundant presence of trace elements, vitamins and enzymes that stimulate digestion and metabolism.

Onion contains a lot of water and has a fair amount of fructose, sugar which, in addition to giving it a certain sweetness, gives it a mild energy function. Proteins and lipids are irrelevant; cholesterol is absent.

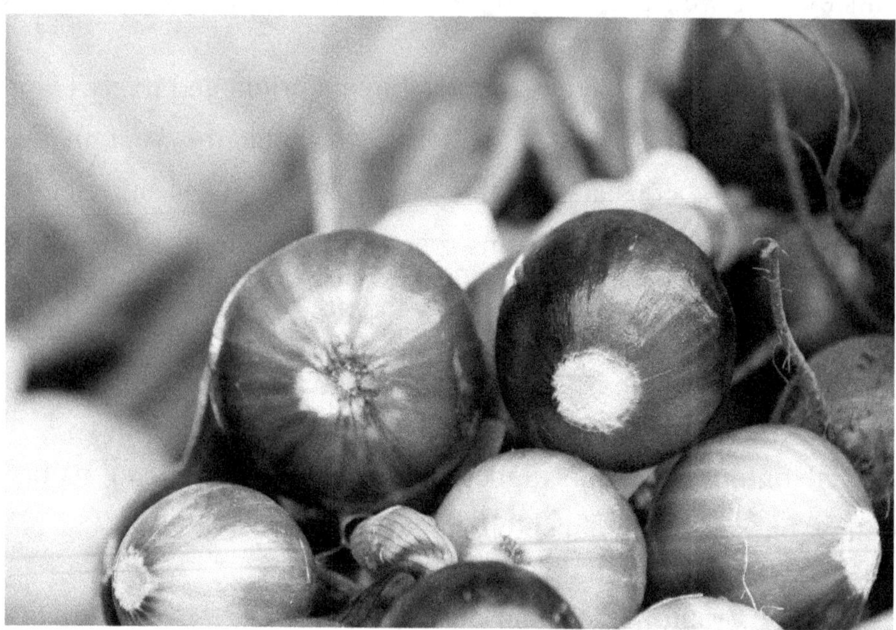

Onion is suitable for most food regimes and, due to the content of some mildly spicy molecules, it can be contraindicated in case of hypersensitivity and / or gastro intestinal diseases such as: stomach acid, gastritis, ulcer, irritable colon, hemorrhoids and anal fissures.

It has no contraindications for overweight and replacement pathologies; on the contrary, it seems to exert a favorable impact on certain metabolic disorders (hypertension, hypercholesterolaemia etc.).

The real "richness" of this vegetable does not show in the energetic, plastic, vitamin or saline nutrients, but in the phytotherapic molecules, most of which have an antioxidant and beneficial function for the metabolism.

It does not contain gluten and lactose, and is accepted by vegetarian and vegan philosophies.

Rocket Salad

Arugula is an annual herbaceous plant belonging to the Brassicaceae family, it has numerous uses, both in the culinary and medical / herbal fields.

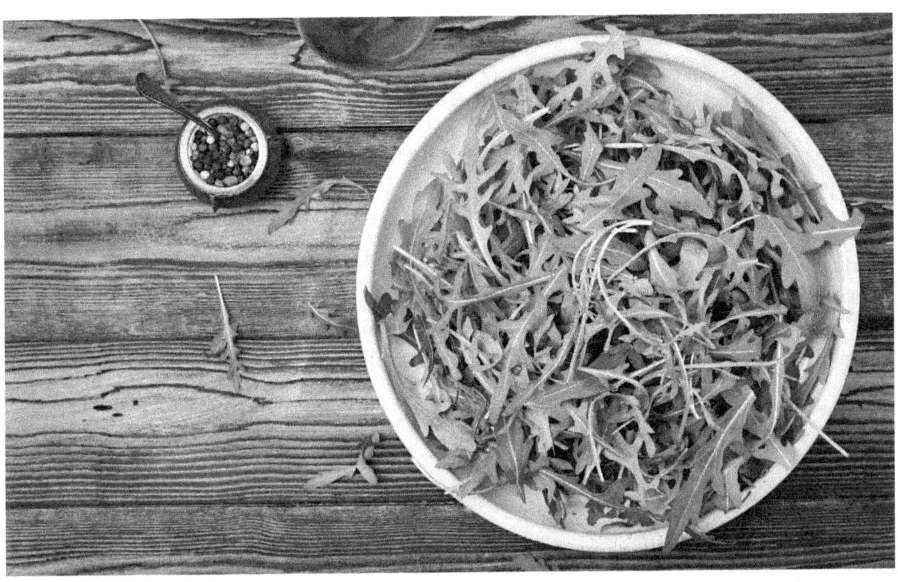

Two types are widespread: the salad rocket and the wild rocket. With the nutrients quercitin and kaempferol they are both two excellent sirtuin activators.

The health aspects of rocket are largely beneficial for our body due to the presence of vitamin C, potassium, iron, calcium and phosphorus. It stimulates appetite and promotes digestion.

Soy

Soy is a legume like beans, chickpeas or lentils, and like all legumes it is rich in B vitamins, iron and potassium. Unlike other legumes, however, soybeans are more digestible and rich in proteins and lipids.

The fruit is a violet colored pod containing 1 to 5 light or dark yellowish seeds depending on the variety. The part used in feeding are the seeds, which contain a high amount of proteins, polyunsaturated lipids and glucosides which include soflavones and saponins. The activating nutrients of sirtuin are daidzein and formononetin.

The interest in the beneficial properties of soy began when some epidemiological studies conducted on Asian populations revealed a lower incidence of some forms of cancer such as breast, colon and prostate cancer. It was also observed that Eastern women had a more serene menopause than Western women and the risk of osteoporosis and cardiovascular disease was reduced.

The existence of a relationship between soy consumption and the reduced incidence of these ailments and pathologies was therefore hypothesized. To confirm this hypothesis, numerous studies were conducted which are still carried out persistently to discover new properties and evaluate their positive effects on health.

The beneficial effects of soy are related to the presence of phytoestrogenie di soflavones which are exploited in phytotherapy. These features mitigate physical ailments associated with menopause such as hot flashes, insomnia, palpitation, osteoporosis and vaginal dryness. These substances have also proven effective in appeasing disturbances in the emotional sphere by reducing anxiety, irritability, depression and humoral instability.

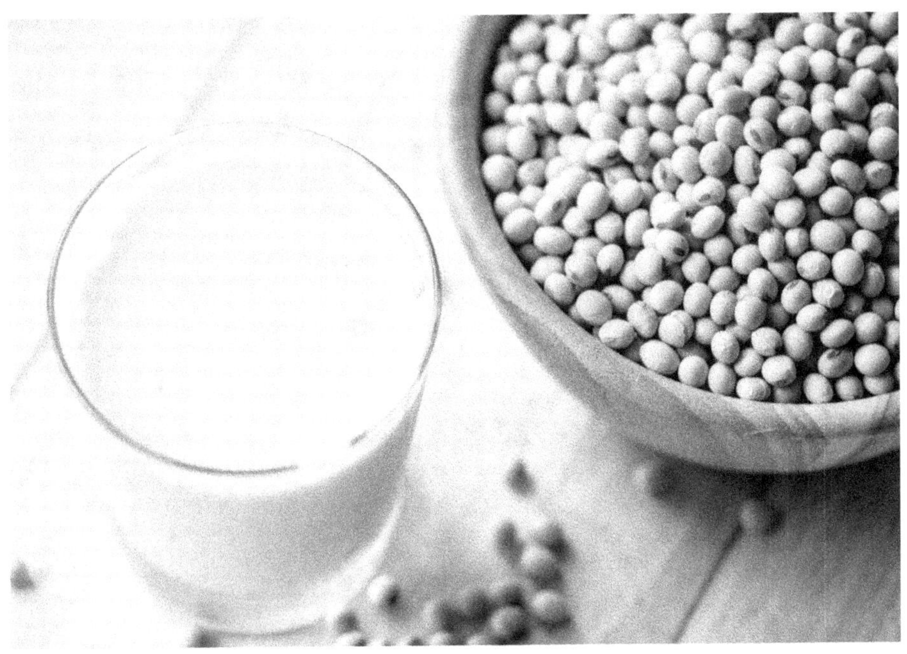

Soy also protects the organism from cardiovascular diseases by lowering blood pressure and cholesterol, improving the elasticity of the arteries and fighting free radicals. However, in high doses, food and derived supplements may not only prove ineffective, but even dangerous to health.

In the nutritional field from soybeans, very rich in proteins and unsaturated fats, many products are obtained such as: milk, tofu, miso, oil, flour and flakes, soy lecithin, soy bread, soy meat, tamari and shoyu.

Miso, made from fermented soybeans, is a traditional Japanese food. In addition to its fantastic beneficial properties for health, the thing that makes it truly indispensable is its wonderful umami flavor, which gives an explosion of taste to your dishes.

Strawberries

The strawberries belong to the Rosaceae family and to the Fragaria genus and are very rich in fisetin, a nutrient activating sirtuine.

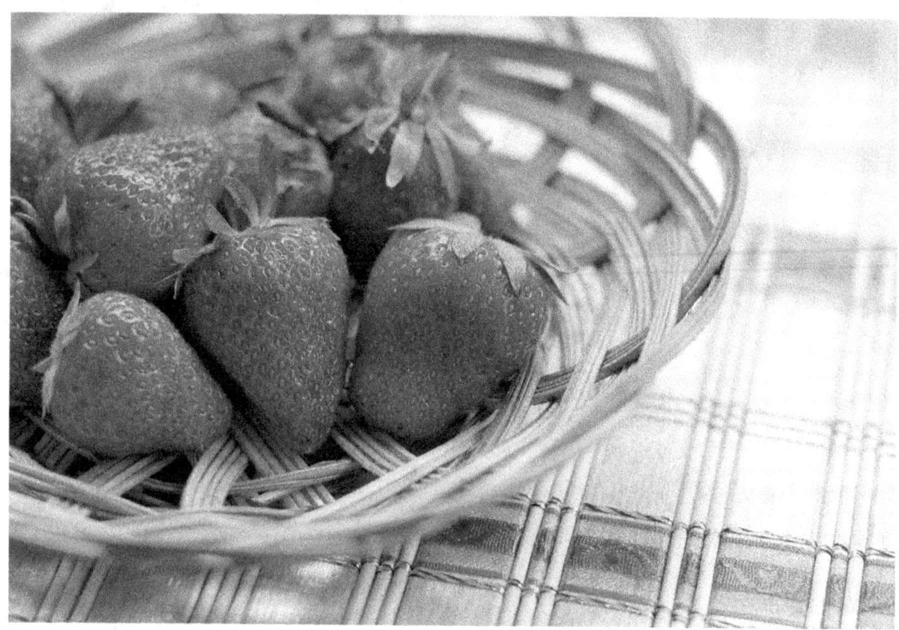

Strawberries have a very low sugar content, 1 teaspoon per 100 g. Added to foods that contain carbohydrates, they help reduce the body's demand for insulin, turning food into a slow-release energy source. They should be an added food of all slimming and healthy diets.

Strawberries are fully ripe fruits and are bright red and yellowish-greenish pigmented. The aroma and sweet taste of strawberries are intense and make them one of the most appreciated and marketed fruits on the whole planet.

Strawberries can be eaten fresh, frozen, dried, in jam, pureed, in syrup and as fruit juice or liquid syrup. In addition, they represent an ingredient widely used in the formulation of ice cream, cakes and desserts.

Of course, everything stems from a myth. Legend says that Mars, jealous of Venus' love for the beautiful Adonis, turned into a wild boar and stabbed him with his fangs during a hunting trip. Venus wept for her beloved and in the place where her tears fell beautiful seedlings of wild strawberries, with the shape of a red heart.

Wild strawberries have been loved since ancient times and have always represented the fruit of love for their shape and lively color. They were consumed in abundance during the Adonìe, spring holidays dedicated to Adonis and love.

In the Middle Ages they became a sinful fruit precisely because it was considered an aphrodisiac. But the strawberry was still known only as wild, wild fruit.

In the gardens, however, they began to be cultivated also for their ornamental value and particular success they had in seventeenth-century France, cared for by illustrious gardeners and introduced into the gardens of the noble houses.

Turmeric

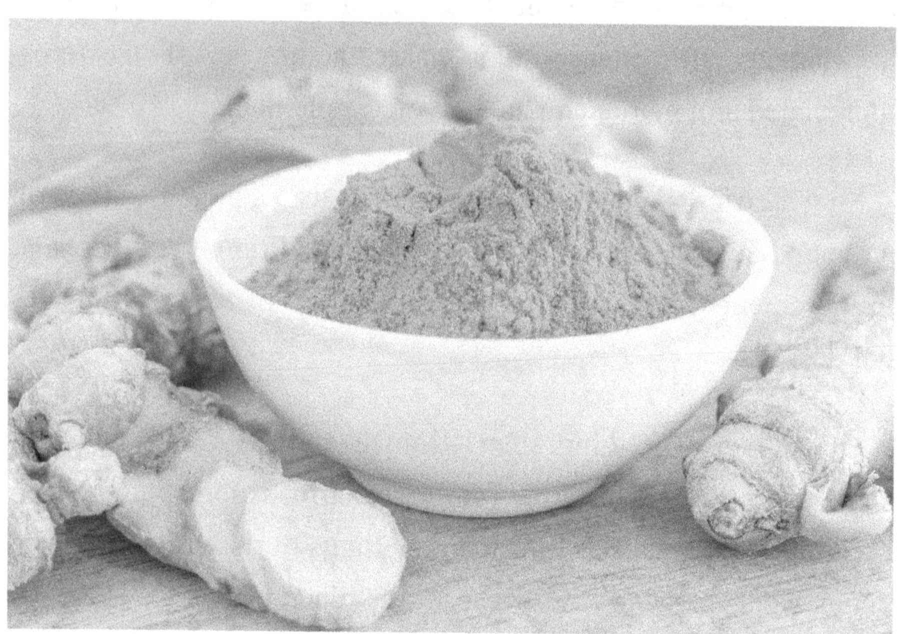

Turmeric is rich in a nutrient, sirtuin activator curcumin. Turmeric is believed to be one of the factors contributing to the lower percentage of cancer patients in India compared to western countries. Studies have shown that a special type of curcumin helps improve cholesterol levels and control blood sugar levels, as well as reducing inflammation. Turmeric has also proven to be an excellent natural pain reliever in cases of osteoarthritis of the knee.

Walnuts

Walnuts are the fruit of the fruit nut plant. Walnut is a plant that falls into the Juglandaceae family. Like pine nuts, almonds, pistachios, walnut is a seed belonging to the group of dried fruit.

Walnuts undermine all traditional beliefs about food. Despite being high in fat and high in calories, it has been widely shown that they contribute to weight loss and improve some metabolic disorders. Walnuts can be eaten fresh or dried and, from the edible part, an oil rich in "good" fats is obtained. Contrary to what most people believe, the fresh and whole fruit of the walnut is fleshy and light green in color. It contains nourishing gallic acid essential for the activation of sirtuin.

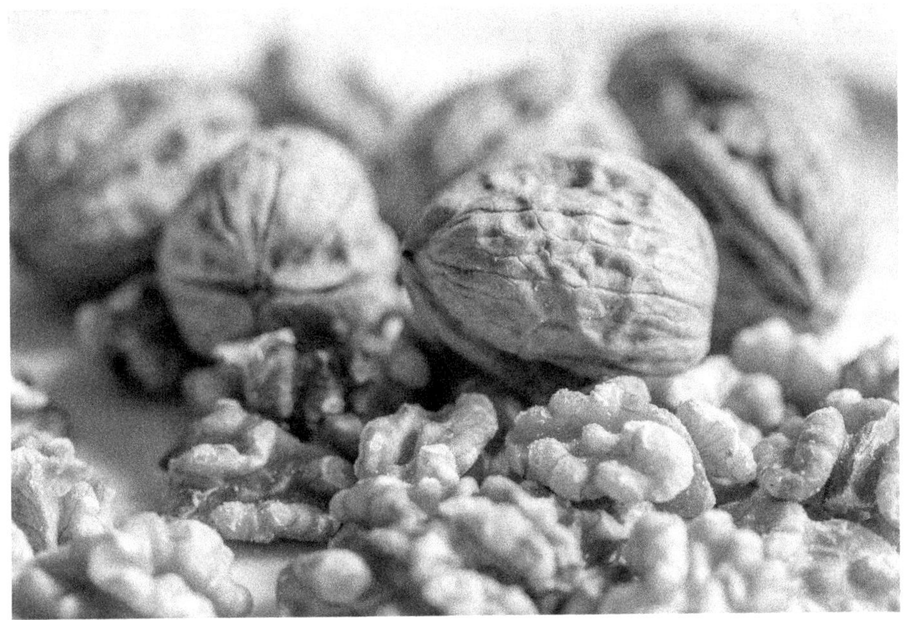

Red Chicory (Radicchio)

Red chicory (also known as radicchio) can be more difficult to find. Alternatively, you can use the yellow one.

Its sour taste adds a particular note to a condiment based on extra virgin olive oil.

Radicchio, rich in vitamins, fiber and mineral salts, conquers for its bitter taste and for the versatility of use in the kitchen

Radicchio is a precious ally for our health because it is a real mine of antioxidants, able to counteract free radicals and cellular aging and also useful against diabetes, constipation and high cholesterol.

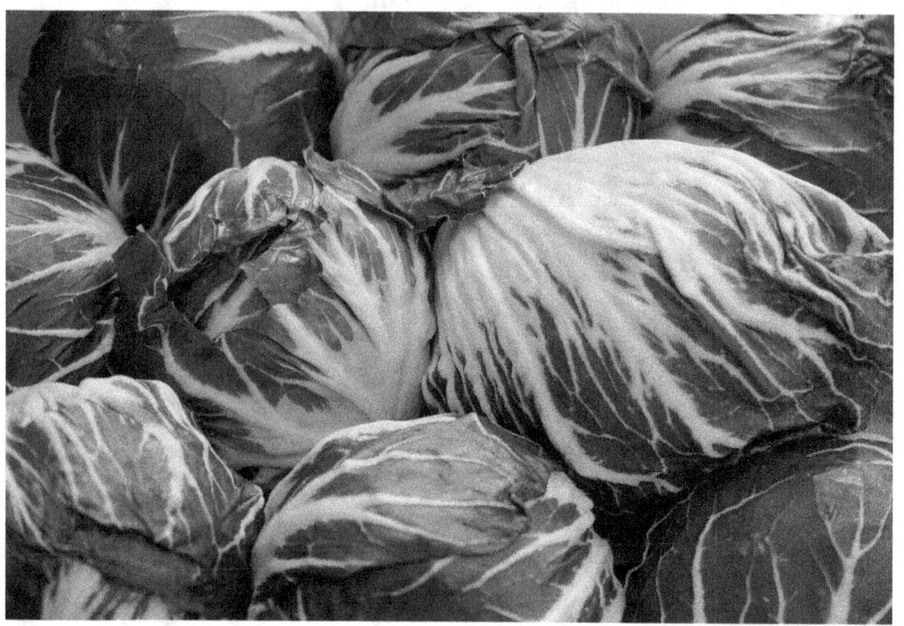

The chicory plant, ChicoriumIntybus, belongs to the Composite family, the same as the chicory group. It is a type of red-violet salad with a bitter taste, thanks to the chicory acid contained in it. It is a vegetable that is found all year round but the best time to consume it is from October until spring, according to the variety.

4. THE SIRT DIET

An original diet

The Sirt diet takes its name from the fact that it is based on sirtuins, enzymatic proteins that help keep the cells of your body healthy. They allow a regular functioning of our body and protect us from various inflammations.

The originality of the sirt diet leverages the use of foods with particular nutrient molecules, polyphenols, which activate enzymatic proteins, sirtuins. They regulate our metabolism, help us burn fat and obviously make us lose weight.

In reality, the diet has been very well known for some time now, also because several characters from the world of entertainment have decided to try it.

However, it is not only for this reason that it is well known. The obvious weight loss that many people have experienced directly and the fact that it is a diet designed to eat everything, has given even more notoriety. In addition, the diet allows the administration of some of the best foods that nature makes available to us. Dark chocolate 85%, red wine, strawberries and berries make us forget that we are undertaking a diet. In addition to the fact that it is a balanced and healthy diet, you lose weight without losing muscle mass.

The diet was developed by 2 renowned dietitians in the UK and Ireland, Aidan Goggins and Glen Matten. The two British nutritionists have studied a program according to which a diet based on certain specific foods can promote rapid weight loss and that the lost pounds do not recover. And if you realize you have gained weight, nothing prevents you from starting again. On the other hand, Sirt foods are a guarantee of genuine, fresh and rich in polyphenols, if used in our daily diet.

Losing weight quickly without fatigue is now a reality. The lean gene diet is an innovative diet. It is based on metabolic regulators, the sirtuins capable of activating a family of genes that exists in each of us. These genes influence our mood, our ability to burn fat and even the mechanisms that regulate our mood and longevity.

The activation of sirtuins, clinically guaranteed by the Sirt diet, produces the same beneficial effects of fasting without the disadvantages. Unlike many other diets, which say what to eliminate, the DietSirt says what to add in our nutrition plan during the diet. This is why it is easier to follow than any other diet.

The Sirt diet is a weight loss program that allows you to lose up to 3 kg in a week while staying healthy and fit.

The Two Phases of the Diet

The diet develops in two stages. The initial, more rigid phase lasts one week and involves limiting calories to 1000 kcal for three days. It is allowed to consume a solid meal a day rich in Sirtfood and three green juices.

During phase 1, it is advisable to reduce the caloric intake and to take every day a juice obtained from cabbage, arugula, green apple, parsley, celery stalks and green tea which can be easily made at home with the help of a centrifuge or an extractor. In this first phase it is possible to lose from 3 to 7 kilograms. It is very important to consume around 1000 calories during the first 3 days.

From the fourth to the seventh day, the heat intake increases to 1500 kcal and includes two green juices and two meals rich in sirtfood per day.

The second phase is known as the "maintenance phase". It lasts 14 days, in which constant weight loss occurs. There are no specific indications regarding the calorie intake, but it is necessary to take a green juice daily and to introduce only Sirt foods in all meals of the day. To maximize results, exercise is also encouraged for about 30 minutes five days a week. We will describe you better this part in the next chapter.

The juices to be made at your choice can include black cabbage, celery, arugula, parsley, green tea and lemon. Solid meals include turkey, chicken, cabbage curry, prawns, buckwheat noodles and onions. They are all foods that are widely used in the preparation of our daily recipes.

The sirt diet is versatile, open, linked to a natural, healthy and appetizing diet. For vegetarians or vegans there are variants with recipes designed specifically. Sirt juices should be drunk at three different times of the day: on waking up, mid-morning and mid-afternoon. A solid meal is recommended for lunch. Very important is to eat three balanced meals rich in sirtfood per day including a green juice.

Diet Sirt, Phase 1: daily menu

• Breakfast: a green juice Sirt

• Snack: a green Sirt juice

• Lunch: a solid, normal or vegan meal.

• Snack: a green Sirt juice

After the first three days of phase 1, solid meals become two, for lunch and dinner.

Generally, you can eat foods that are high in protein and low in fat. Among the meat recipes, you can choose for example chicken with red onion and black cabbage, turkey with cauliflower couscous, turkey escalope with capers and parsley. For fish dishes such as stir-fried salmon fillet, stir-fried prawns or baked marinated cod. Recipes of side dishes, light and tasty, prepared with beans, lentils, aubergines cut into wedges and cooked in the oven, waldorf salad or red onions.

And as a dessert, the delicious and healthy strawberries, with a very high content of sirtuins. Also remember that 15-20g of dark chocolate are allowed every day.

Green Juices Recipes

It is a completely natural juice and characterized by its green color given by its ingredients. This drink has the greatest ability to purify and satiate. Juices during the diet should be consumed 1 hour before the solid meal or 2 hours after. And another rule, you must have dinner by 7:00pm.

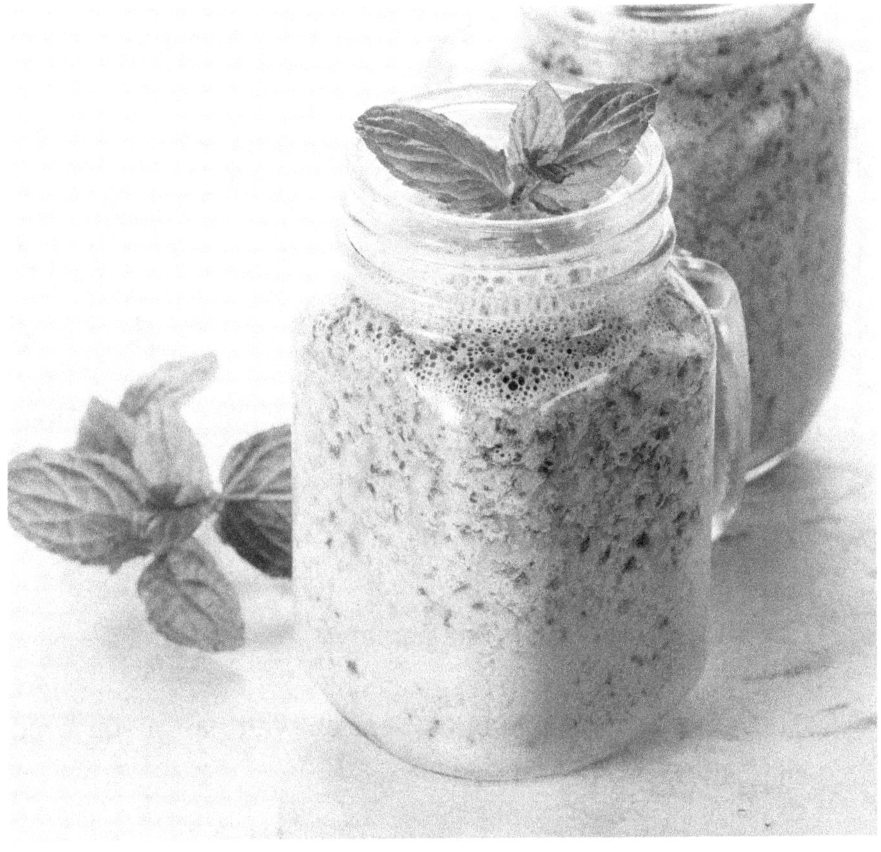

As we have seen, it is a diet that, above all in the first days, is based on a miraculous green juice. A completely natural drink that is combined first with one and then with two solid meals.

Green juice is an important part of the diet, because it has the ability to cleanse and detoxify, and will be the main character in the first week of the Sirt program.

You have to prepare it three times a day and you will need a centrifuge and a kitchen scale, because the ingredients are listed by weight. Juice must always be prepared when consuming it. The recipe is below:

Ingredients

- 75g of curly kale
- 30g of rocket
- 5g of parsley
- 150g of green celery with leaves
- 1/2 green apple
- 1/2 lemon juice
- 1/2 teaspoon matcha tea

Preparation

1. Centrifuge kale, rocket and parsley.

2. Add grated celery and apple; enrich with half a squeezed lemon and half a teaspoon of matcha tea.

3. Drink immediately so you don't miss out on the valuable benefits of nutrients.

A Typical Week

The menu that we will provide you is purely informative as your nutritionist or dietician will adapt it according to your singular needs. Obviously each person is characterized by their own clinical history, and it is precisely based on their general health condition that nutrition experts can develop a diet that meets their needs.

Monday:

3 portions of green juice

- *Breakfast*: a glass of water accompanied by a cup of coffee or tea + a cup of green juice (to be prepared at our choice).

- *Lunch:* a single portion of green juice

- *Snack:* a piece of dark chocolate 10 g

- *Dinner:* buckwheat integrated through pasta or rice, accompanied by chicken and vegetables of our choice.

- *After dinner*: a piece of dark chocolate 10 g

Tuesday:

3 portions of green juice

- *Breakfast:* a glass of water accompanied by a cup of coffee or tea + a cup of green juice (to be prepared at our choice).

- *Lunch*: two green juices to be taken before dinner

- *Snack*: a piece of dark chocolate

- *Dinner*: couscous, spelled, barley etc. with vegetables + chicken or fish (shrimp)

- *After dinner*: a piece of dark chocolate

Wednesday:

3 portions of green juice (or centrifuged)

- *Breakfast*: a glass of water accompanied by a cup of coffee or tea + a cup of green juice (to be prepared at our choice).

- *Lunch*: two green juices to be taken before dinner

- *Snack*: a piece of dark chocolate

- *Dinner*: quantity vegetables + chicken or fish

- *After dinner*: a piece of dark chocolate

Thursday:

2 portions of green juice (or centrifuged)

- *Breakfast*: a glass of water accompanied by a cup of coffee or tea + a cup of green juice (to be prepared at our choice).

- *Lunch*: Muesli

- *Snack*: a green juice before dinner

- *Dinner*: vegetable soup of our choice

Friday:

green juice: 2 times a day

- *Breakfast*: a glass of water + tea or espresso + a cup of green juice
- *Lunch*: buckwheat salad with vegetables;
- *Snack*: a green juice before dinner;
- *Dinner*: fish or meat with vegetables and baked potatoes.

Saturday:

green juice: 2 times a day

- *Breakfast*: a bowl of muesli cereals accompanied by a cup of green juice
- *Lunch*: omelette and bacon;
- *Snack*: a cup of green juice;
- *Dinner*: chicken, walnuts and parsley + a red onion + tomato salad.

Sunday:

green juice: 2 times a day

- *Breakfast*: a glass of water, tea or coffee + a cup of green juice;
- *Lunch*: salad accompanied by grilled fish or chicken;
- *Snack*: a cup of green juice;
- *Dinner*: fish or meat cooked with a drizzle of red wine and plenty of salad and vegetables.

Contraindications of the Sirt Diet

Is the Sirt Diet effective? The problem is that there is not much evidence to support the fact that the sirt diet has an effective scientific effect. However, there is a pilot study conducted. The experiment involved 39 participants in the fitness center conducted by the 2 dieticians, authors of the Sirt diet. However, the results of this study were published in the book "Sirt, the lean gene diet".

For a week, the participants followed the diet and exercised daily physical activity.

At the end of the week, participants lost an average of 3.2 kg and maintained or even gained muscle mass. However, it appears that the method has not been tested and documented in the long term. Moreover, limiting the calorie intake to 1,000 calories, sustaining a physical training and eliminating the almost all carbohydrates, following the first phase of the Sirt diet, will certainly lead to weight loss.

This study did not follow participants after the first week to see if they had gained weight afterwards. In addition, with the Sirt diet, aimed at activating the "weight loss genes", foods that activate the metabolism are assumed, while pretending to be sated, thus creating a sort of deception for the body. This diet is likely to help you lose a few pounds at first, but will likely return as soon as the diet is over. On the other hand, adding Sirt foods to your usual long-term diet can be a good idea. In this case, however, you can also avoid the diet and start a new food education based on the consumption of Sirt foods. As for disease prevention, three weeks are probably not long enough to have a measurable long-term impact.

are probably not long enough to have a measurable long-term impact.

5. SOME RECIPES

Solid Food Recipes

The Sirt diet includes specific foods and we would like to show some recipes to make at home. Some recipes to prepare, after consulting with your doctor who will be able to evaluate your health and the most suitable diet, to make you lose weight in total safety.

Chicken with Red Onion and Black Cabbage

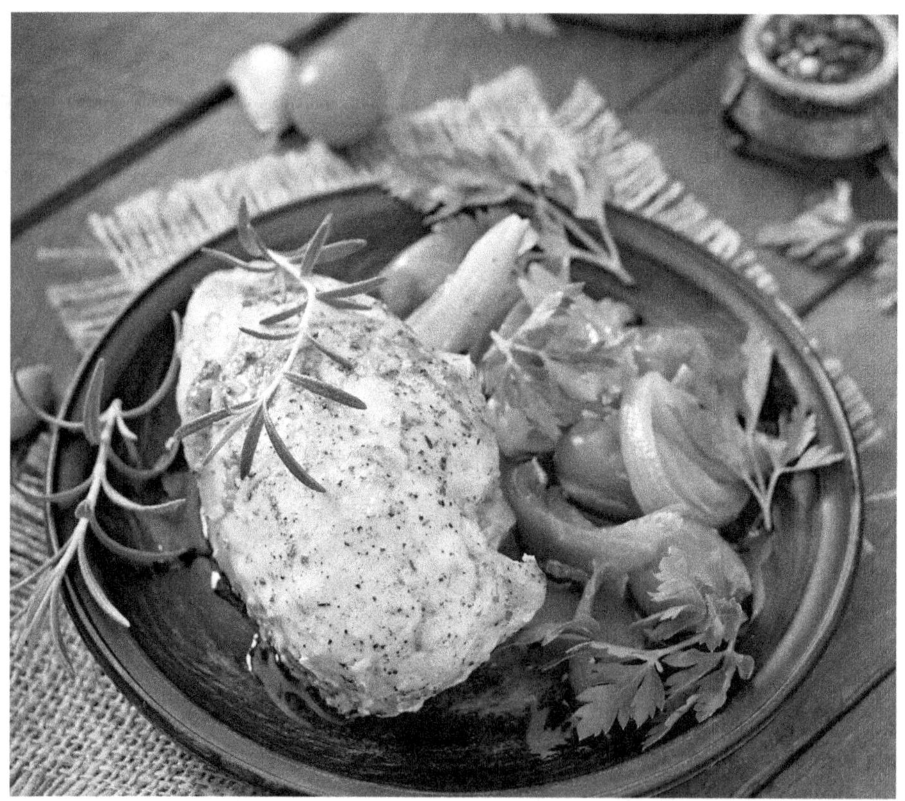

Ingredients

- 120g of chicken breast
- 130g of tomatoes
- 1 chilli pepper
- 1 tablespoon of capers
- 5g of parsley
- lemon juice
- 2 tbsp. Extra virgin olive oil
- 2 teaspoons of turmeric
- 50g of cabbage
- 20g of red onion
- 1 teaspoon fresh ginger
- 50g of buckwheat

Preparation

Marinate the chicken breast for 10 minutes with 1/4 of lemon juice, 1 tablespoon of extra virgin olive oil and 1 teaspoon of turmeric powder.

Cut 130g of chopped tomatoes, remove the inside, season with Bird's Eye pepper, 1 tablespoon of capers, 1 teaspoon of turmeric and one of extra virgin olive oil, 1/4 of lemon juice and 5g of parsley chopped.

Fry the chicken breast, dripped from the marinade, on a high flame for one minute on each side, then put it in the oven for about 10 minutes at 220 ° C.

Let it rest covered with aluminum foil.

Steam the chopped kale for 5 minutes.

Sauté a red onion, a teaspoon of grated fresh ginger and a teaspoon of extra virgin olive oil; add the cooked cabbage and cook for a minute on the fire.

Boil the buckwheat with a teaspoon of turmeric, drain and serve with chicken, tomatoes and chopped cabbage.

Turkey With Cauliflower CousCous

Ingredients

- 150g of turkey
- 150g of cauliflower
- 40g of red onion
- 1 teaspoon fresh ginger
- 1 bird's eye pepper
- 1 clove of garlic
- 3 tablespoons of extra virgin olive oil
- 2 teaspoons of turmeric
- 30g of dried tomatoes
- 10g of parsley

- dried sage to taste

- 1 tablespoon of capers

- 1/4 of fresh lemon juice

Preparation

Blend the raw cauliflower tops and cook them in a teaspoon of extra virgin olive oil, garlic, red onion, chilli pepper, ginger and a teaspoon of turmeric.

Leave to flavor for a minute, then add the chopped sun-dried tomatoes and 5g of parsley over the heat.

Season the turkey slice with a teaspoon of extra virgin olive oil, the dried sage and cook it in another teaspoon of extra virgin olive oil.

Once ready, season with a tablespoon of capers, 1/4 of lemon juice, 5g of parsley, a tablespoon of water and add the cauliflower.

Tips

*Chocolate**

Choose dark chocolate with 85% cocoa, rich in antioxidants, it has a low glycemic index.

*Green tea***

Known because it is so good for our body, green tea contributes to the loss of fat, preserving the muscles. Choose the Matcha variety and drink it with the addition of a little lemon juice, which increases the absorption of the nourishing activators of sirtuins.

*Chili pepper****

To spice up your dishes, use Bird'sEye (also called Thai) chili pepper, which is very rich in sirtuine.

You can use it at least three times a week.

Coffee

You can drink 3-4 cups a day being careful not to overdo it with sugar and avoid adding milk.

Buckwheat Salad

Buckwheat salad is a tasty first course, also excellent cold and gluten-free. It can be customized with the ingredients you prefer and never disappoints. Here is the recipe.

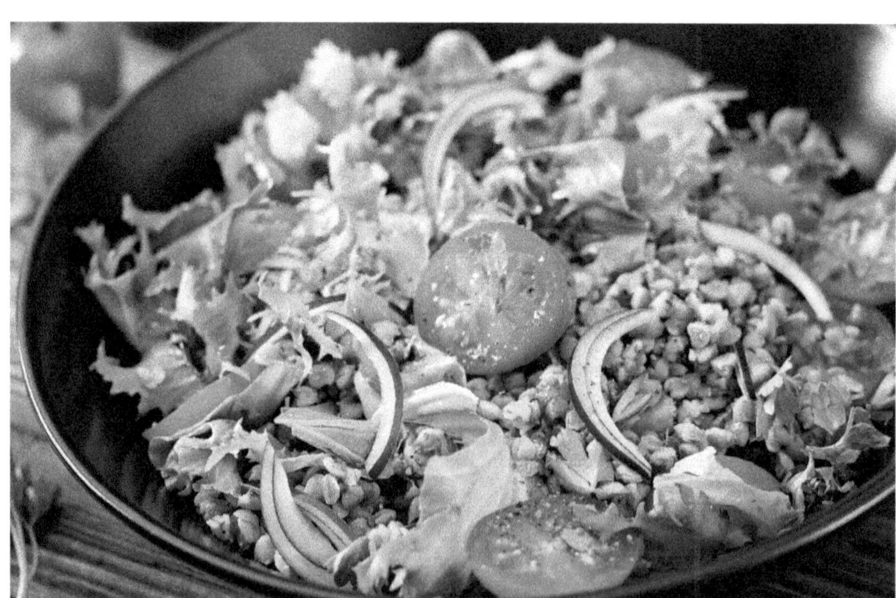

Prep.: 15 min

Cooking: 25min

Total time: 40 min

Doses for: 4 people

Ingredients

- 150g of buckwheat

- 150g of frozen beans (or fresh if in season)

- 1 courgette

- 1 carrot

- 1 clove of garlic

- 20g of salted capers

- 1 handful of sesame seeds (or sunflower)

- Some basil leaves

- 1 teaspoon hot pepper

- 1 teaspoon balsamic vinegar to taste

- Extra virgin olive oil to taste

- Salt to taste.

You cook!

First, blanch the beans in abundant salted water until they are cooked but al dente. Peel and cut the carrot into cubes half a centimeter thick. Do the same with courgette.

Cook the vegetables.

In a non-stick pan, heat a drizzle of extra virgin olive oil with the garlic clove. As soon as it has taken a little color and flavored the oil, remove it and add the chopped carrots. Cook for about 5 minutes, then add the courgettes and cook on a high flame for another 10 minutes, being careful not to burn the vegetables. A few minutes after the end of cooking, add the broad beans and season with the chilli pepper, capers, sesame seeds and coarsely chopped basil by hand. Stir to mix all the ingredients well and season with salt.

Cook the wheat.

Boil the buckwheat in abundant salted water, then drain it al dente and season it with the vegetables. Add the balsamic vinegar and mix before serving.

Buckwheat salad can be kept in an airtight container and in the refrigerator for a couple of days.

Farro with Vegetables and Chicken

Farro with chicken and vegetables is a light dish and at the same time rich in flavor and nutritional properties, it is suitable for all seasons and ideal for a light and detoxifying diet. Farro is one of the cereals whose cultivation dates back to the most ancient temples, it has been consumed since the Neolithic period. It was the main basis of the diet of the ancient Romans and was mainly used to prepare bread, focaccia and polenta. Spelled with chicken and vegetables is an excellent single dish, which can be eaten both hot and cold.

Ingredients:

- 320g of spelled,
- 2 courgettes,
- 3 carrots,
- 2 potatoes,
- 150g of green beans,
- 150g of peas,
- 300g of chicken,
- 1 onion,
- 2 cloves of garlic,
- Extra virgin olive oil,
- Parsley,
- Salt to taste.

Preparation

Wash the spelled and cook it in boiling salted water for 25 minutes.

Wash and cut the vegetables.

In a pan, brown the onion and the garlic cloves minced in 3 tablespoons of oil, add the diced chicken, brown it, sprinkle with a little white wine, let it evaporate, add 1 ladle of broth, salt to taste and cook for 20 minutes.

At this point add the vegetables and continue cooking for 10 minutes.

Drain the spelled and add it to the chicken and vegetables. Mix and cook for a few minutes over low heat, add chopped parsley and serve.

Vegetable Soup

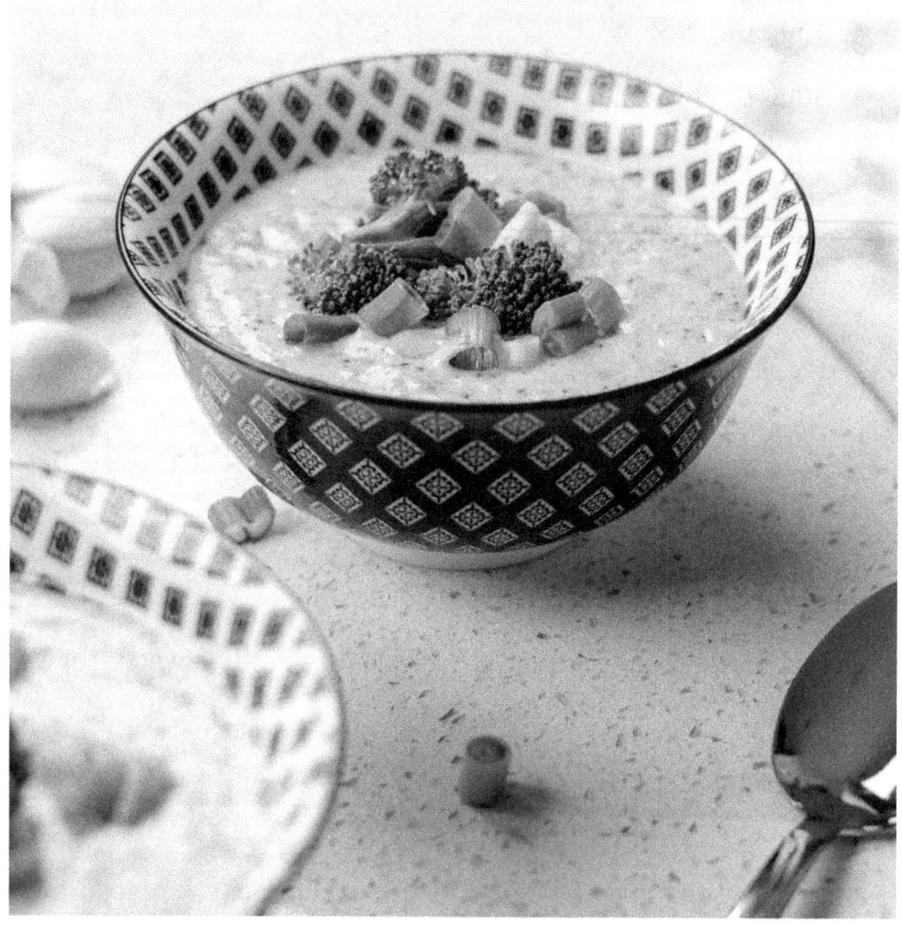

If you think of a healthy dish, a recipe immediately comes to mind: the vegetable soup. It is a recipe that can change its appearance depending on the season. Cold in summer and warm in winter, it changes according to the scents and colors of the vegetables that the garden offers. Today we offer a winter version, excellent to be enjoyed hot and steaming, which will surely be able to warm you up when the weather forces you to take refuge in front of the fireplace. The preparation of this vegetable minestrone is somewhat simple but rather long and laborious, due to the cleaning and cutting of the ingredients that compose it. We guarantee, however, that it is really worth taking the time to taste this simple first course of vegetables because it is a recipe capable of combining goodness and authenticity. Make way for vegetables in the kitchen: today we prepare a delicious vegetable soup!

Ingredients:

- Carrots 80g

- Red onions 80g

- White courgettes 150g

- Potatoes 330g

- Salt to taste

- Black pepper to taste

- Celery 60g

- Auburn tomatoes 350g

- Borlotti beans 200g

- Clean pumpkin 250g

- Extra virgin olive oil 50g

- Leeks 150g

- Clean cauliflower 300g

- Peas 200g

- Rosemary 1 sprig

- Laurel 2 leaves

- Water to taste

To prepare the vegetable soup, start by washing and drying the vegetables. Then take the pumpkin and remove the outer skin with a knife with a large blade. Remove the seeds and internal filaments with the help of a spoon. Then cut it into slices of equal thickness and then into cubes of about 1cm on the side. Wash and peel the courgettes, cut them into slices, and cut them into cubes. Then shell the beans, then from the latter cut into cubes. Proceed with the tomatoes: remove the stalk and cut them into slices. Then also reduce the tomatoes into cubes. Also finely chop celery. To finish, tie the sprigs of rosemary with bay leaves to create an aromatic bunch. Now all the ingredients for preparing the vegetable minestrone are ready. Pour the oil into a large pot with lid carrots, celery, onion and leek and brown gently for about ten minutes, stirring often. Once the sautéed vegetables are softened add the fragrant bunch and pour the beans.

Cover with water: it will have to cover the vegetables by an inch. Wait for the boiling point and cook for 2 minutes. Add the pumpkin and repeat the same procedure: add water until it covers by an inch, wait for the boil to resume and cook for 2 minutes. Same thing with the potatoes, and to follow with the cauliflower.

Cover with more water, put the lid and cook 25 minutes from the resumption of the boil. After 25 minutes add courgettes, peas and tomatoes, add water if necessary, season with salt and pepper and cook again 2-3 minutes after boiling again.

Smoked Salmon Salad

The smoked salmon salad is a tasty appetizer that brings together different flavors and textures, which bind wonderfully well. The succulent and sour sweetness of the oranges, the vaguely herbaceous flavor and the creaminess of the avocado and the smoked touch of salmon combined in a single dish.

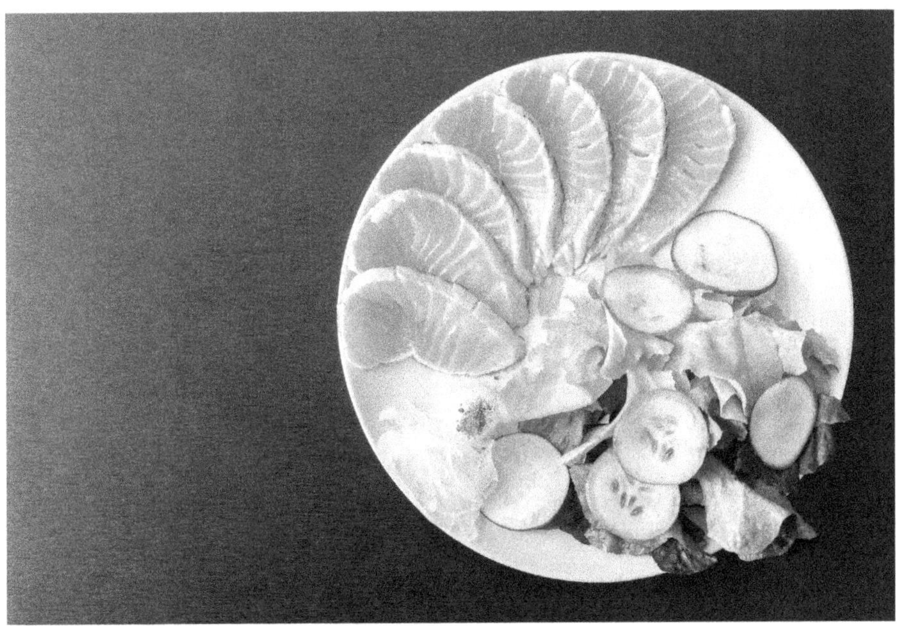

As for avocado, I suggest you get one from California, of the species called Hass, with dark and wrinkled skin: they are much tastier and buttery than those of Florida, which are instead larger and with a smoother and light green color. To verify that it is ripe at the right point, you will have to rely on the touch, gently pressing your thumb on the fruit: if it is very hard, it means that it is still unripe and therefore must be kept a couple of days out of the fridge, in a paper bag together with an apple, so it will ripen faster. The right avocado for this preparation is such if by pressing on the peel the fruit is elastic but no groove remains, this means that it is ripe but not excessively soft and therefore perfect for cutting into pieces.

To prepare the Smoked Salmon Salad, start by taking care of the orange, then peel it raw using a sharp knife: to do this you must remove all the peel and the white part, revealing the fruit pulp. During this operation, place it on a small bowl, to collect the juice that will come out. Also remove the skin that covers the wedges, the seeds, if there are, cut them into slices and put them in a bowl. Keep the juice that has spilled from the orange aside.

Separately prepare the dressing: add a drizzle of olive oil and a generous pinch of salt to the orange juice, then mix well. If the orange juice is low, you can add more or you can add a little lemon or lime juice.

6. PHYSICAL ACTIVITY

Sports and Daily Commitments

The commitment to exercise regularly may appear incompatible with the rhythms and lifestyle habits of many people. It is not easy to cut time, but with stubbornness it is possible to succeed. It is important to play sports to dispose of what we eat.

Surely the first step is to become aware of the importance of physical activity. A more detailed handbook could help us choose the most suitable solution for our needs.

If you have time available early in the morning before breakfast or in the evening before dinner, a nice ride would be ideal. Before training it is a good habit to have a cup of matcha tea which increases thermogenesis which allows the consumption of more energy.

For those who have little time but goodwill with small daily tricks, they will almost unwittingly do their physical activity. If we really cannot avoid using the car, we try to park it far from the place where we have to go, in order to walk at least 5 minutes. If we use public transport, we can get off one or two stops earlier. If we live on the penthouse, we use our foot. Going on foot is a good habit to acquire, instead of hitchhiking the car to get around.

For those who have a lot of time but little will, a method that can help overcome laziness could be to be followed by a personal trainer. Or do physical activity with more motivated friends. Having a dog can also be a great incentive to go for a walk.

Doing exercises with the help of a web tutorial, doing yoga, fitness or CrossFit are all training programs designed for those who do not have time to go to the gym and want to take some time to start exercising again.

The most difficult cases are those of those who have little time and little will. These are the cases that, like all difficult ones, should be seen as a challenge. It is appropriate to make a bet on ourselves. Maybe by proposing to try to do physical activity for a limited period, because we know habits need to be changed slowly, especially the more deeply rooted ones.

If you change your mentality, you change your physique. The greatest gratification will come when only for one's own merit will it be to be fit, full of energy and planning. Losing weight means taking care of yourself and returning to feeling good, waking up with a smile and being energetic all day. It's just a matter of desire, time, mind and organization.

So, we find the exercise that best suits our abilities and needs, and we try to do it regularly and consistently.

Rules to Keep in Mind

- ✓ Before embarking on any type of physical activity, it is better to undergo a sports-medical examination.

✓ Avoid activities with a strong joint impact, which can stress the joints excessively.

✓ You prefer sports such as swimming, cycling or walking. Sports that require certain steps of graduality are the only ones capable of promoting calcium metabolism and counteracting osteoporosis.

✓ Do aerobic activity. It begins gradually with 10-minute sessions, interspersed with short breaks. Incrementally for 20 minutes, 30 minutes.

✓ Include some stretching exercises, in moderation, to improve your flexibility.

✓ Avoid training during the hottest hours of the day in summer or in too humid or cold environments in winter.

✓ Drink at least 2 liters of water a day and during training, with small frequent sips.

✓ Choose flat surfaces for jogging, with appropriate footwear to avoid inflammation or muscle pain.

✓ Don't limit yourself to just sitting in the gym or your daily sports minutes. Take advantage of every opportunity to move.

Eliminate Excess Fat

Those who follow the sirt diet should perform also physical activity. This is valid for everybody. The movement stimulates the activation of sirtuins for the benefit of health. Moreover, being overweight increases the risk of contracting serious illnesses.

Obesity, both for young people and for adults is one of the most important diseases of western society. It is associated with cardiovascular diseases, heart attack, stroke, hypertension, type 2 diabetes and debilitating diseases such as osteoarthritis, gout, and metabolic syndrome.

People often go on a diet because they believe that eating less and suffering from hunger is the only way to lose weight and stay healthy. Very questionable behavior. Obese people who really want to lose weight and enjoy good health must necessarily act on adequate nutrition and gradual physical activity.

Losing 1 kg of pure fat mass with a low calorie diet is particularly difficult. Normally, a kilo of body mass is made up largely of 75-80% of fat and the rest 20-25% of muscles and corresponds to about 7000 kcal.

One kilo of weight, of pure fat mass, in energetic terms values 9000 calories (kcal). If then, it is taken into consideration that the body tries to conserve fat as much as possible as it considers it an energy reserve, then one understands the difficulty in disposing of too much fat.

The most logical solution to burn excess fat is possible only if you adopt a balanced low-calorie diet, accompanied by a good level of exercise.

A non-low-calorie and balanced diet in sirt nutrients allows you to eliminate fat mass more and more, only if the diet is associated with an adequate sport program, on the contrary, the muscles will suffer.

The low-calorie diet, low in carbohydrates and proteins, lowers the metabolism by about 40 kcal, for every kilo of lean mass lost. After a certain period of fasting, when the subjects return to eat normally, the body's metabolism, no longer stressed for the loss of lean body mass, will be slower. The lost pounds will be taken up with the interest. Drastic, unbalanced or monotonous diets are the main cause of yo-yo syndrome, characterized by a very rapid drop and weight recovery. Physical activity, it is good to reiterate it, not only helps to preserve lean body mass more, but also tones and strengthens the muscles. In addition, it reduces blood pressure, triglycerides, visceral adipose tissue, bad cholesterol and muscle tone.

Obviously, constancy and regularity are needed to obtain benefits from physical activity. Three hours of concentrated Sunday activities are less effective than those that will be spread over several days of the week. Then, another factor not to be underestimated is to opt for physical activities that provide some satisfaction. Our exercise must be fun, maybe even varied to induce those who are easily bored to avoid stress.

Tone the Lean Mass

It is wrong to focus only on aerobic exercises, leaving out the anaerobic aspect and toning. Spending many hours on a treadmill certainly promotes fat consumption. However, the excess of excessive fat loss predisposes our body to the release of the stress hormone, cortisol. It slows down the metabolism, accelerates water retention and the perception of the feeling of general tiredness. In fact, one feels very tired and the body will be less toned.

A correct training card, must take into account the basic muscle composition, for women in particular, of the targeted training needs for legs, buttocks and abdominals, to ensure good toning for a pleasant aesthetic.

At the level of muscle growth, men and women share the same structure, the obvious difference lies in the production of natural testosterone, which obviously is higher in men and allows them to increase mass in a much more considerable way.

To obtain the desired results, therefore, we must integrate training with exercises that use weights and machines. Strength training, with weights, barbells and kettlebells, studied on individual needs, is the right way to tone your muscles.

Power-ups with tools are important for developing lean mass over fat. The calorie expenditure associated with tonic muscles is higher than the fat mass. It is possible to eat the same, following a sirt diet, but consuming more calories per day. Muscle development and endurance allow bones to remain compact, useful for preventing osteoporosis.

Fitness for Women

Women choose fitness to keep fit, to lose a few extra pounds and, more and more frequently, to feel good about themselves. Taking care of your body's health with sport is not easy. So much so that you can run into multiple mistakes. One of the most common mistakes is to avoid warming up before starting training. This practice is very important, because it allows the body to enter temperature. For toned abs it is enough to dedicate yourself as for the other muscles, two or three times a week, with a couple of sets done carefully and slowly. It is not advisable to practice long series of exercises, otherwise the result could be prominent abdomen and possible damage to the back and posture

To obtain a harmonic body we must not underestimate any part of our body. Stretch and squat push-ups and assume fundamental importance for the toning of all parts of the body. Push-ups, in particular, represent one of the few exercises that, in one gesture, set muscles in the whole body in motion.

The endorphins, after a training session, make us feel exhausted but enthusiastic, to the point that we can't wait to go back to the gym. In doing so, there is a risk of straining the muscle with harmful injuries

Rest, in fact, is as important as training. It is good to give a certain muscle band a break of at least 48.

Breathing is important, like rest, if you want to maximize the effectiveness of training. Constancy is the key to obtaining the desired results thanks to sports and fitness. The ideal would soon be to find a balance that allows you to combine family, work, commitments and training. The goal can only be achieved if this is sustainable in the long run.

Targeted Exercises

Training in a wrong way has as a first effect the failure to achieve the goal we have set. If we want to make our body more harmonious, toned and lean, and we don't expect the right rules, we probably won't see the change we want.

A wrong load, excessive training intensity, a concentrated effort on some limbs or muscles increases the chances of obtaining microtraumas or other injuries. Training will soon become a source of stress and frustration, if we do not take note of our mistakes, with the only result of letting us abandon our program.

It is easy to get caught up in enthusiasm and choose to train starting from easy exercises setting your own goals which are, of course, subjective and personal.

Aerobic activities stimulate the body to use large quantities of oxygen and help the muscles and encourage the consumption of calories.

For women who aspire to have a harmonious body and want to tone their body, it would be advisable to practice a complete workout, even at the time of music, which includes push-ups, bends, stretches and exercises with small dumbbells and kettlebells.

Various Exercises

To work completely on the whole musculature, with harmonious effects on an aesthetic level and health benefits a weekly training session for women, must take into account the variability of the weights and the intensity of the training. Contrary to what many women think, it will not be some exercise commensurate with their body to disfigure the female body with man exercises. In any case, weight training is essential alternating with aerobics. The equipment will be suitable for those who use them are beginners or habitual to these practices.

Below is an example of a program that requires continuous work, in order to burn the largest number of energy. Obviously, it is enough to choose only one activity per session.

- treadmill for cardio exercise - 10 minutes

- oblique crunch for abs - 3 sets x 12 reps per side

- crunch on flat bench for abs - 3 sets x 15 reps

- pelvis twists - 3 sets x max repetitions in 1 minute

- adductor machine for inner thigh - 3 sets x 15 reps

- abductor machine for external thigh - 3 sets x 15 reps

- leg press for legs - 3 sets x 12 reps

- step for cardio exercise - 15 minutes

- elliptical trainer for cardio exercise - 10 minutes

- presses on an inclined bench for the chest - 3 sets for 15 repetitions

- triceps with dumbbell behind - 3 sets for 12 reps

- lat machine ahead for the backbones - 3 sets for 12 reps

- exercise bike for cardio exercise - 5 minutes

Program why you want to work on gaining muscle mass, using body building machines. You can start using light loads.

- treadmill or stepper or elliptical - 10 minutes

- abdominal machine for the abdominals - 25 kg of weight for 2 sets and 10 reps (to be increased up to 35 kg of weight for 3 sets with 15 reps)

- abdominal crunch - 2 sets for 12 reps

Leg press for legs - 40 kg weight for 2 sets and 10 reps (to be increased up to 55 kg for 3 sets and 12 reps)

- gluteus machine for the buttocks - 10 kg of weight for 2 sets and 10 reps (to be increased up to 25 kg for 3 sets and 15 reps)

- adductor machine for inner thigh - 15 kg of weight for 2 sets and 12 reps (to be increased up to 55 kg for 3 sets and 15 reps)

- shoulder press for shoulders - 10 kg of weight for 2 sets and 10 reps (to be increased up to 15 kg for 3 sets and 12 reps)

- triceps at the top cables - 10 kg weight for 2 sets and 10 repetitions (to be increased up to 20 kg for 3 sets and 12 repetitions)

- chest press for the chest - 10 kg of weight for 2 sets and 10 reps (to be increased up to 25 kg for 3 sets and 15 reps)

Back pulley - 10 kg weight for 2 sets and 10 reps (to be increased up to 15 kg for 3 sets and 15 reps)

• treadmill - 5 minutes.

This training of about 3 sessions per week will be ideal if the training is carried out in a constant and gradual way.

7. SIRT DIET AND INTERMITTENT FASTING

A food program

The Sirt diet could be combined perfectly with the intermittent fasting, because the very principle of this diet is to lose weight on the basis of energy consumption. In fact, the intermittent fasting is a diet that alternates periods of eating and fasting. It can be viewed as a nutritional approach rather than a real diet. In practice, at same level of calories embodied, it is possible to burn more energy by consuming meals with lower frequency than usual. This prevents hunger and accelerates the metabolic process. By skipping meals, it is possible to create a caloric deficit and then lose weight, as long as one does compensate for fasting periods with foods rich in sugar or fat. Obviously, this system works only if the caloric amount and the nutritional breakdown are balanced.

The protocol includes 3 daily meals, 1 training session and a fasting period of 16 hours.

- 1st meal to be eaten as soon as one gets up: protein source and carbohydrates with medium-low glycemic index, low fat.

- 2nd meal - breakfast: complete

- Physical activity

- 3rd meal, to be carried out immediately after training. Complete lunch.

- Fasting period from 13:00 or 15:00 until the following morning.

Clearly, the program is to be adapted to the subjective lifestyle. Although the fasting window is respected, meals cannot be eaten without limits. Also, in order to maximize the results of slimming and gaining muscle mass, it is always necessary to perform the right physical activity.

Some advice to start

Trying intermittent fasting means to follow specific tips. It is important to make sure that the diet is healthy and balanced. Eat high-fiber foods to satisfy your hunger, fruits, vegetables, legumes and sirt foods, high-quality proteins, fish, soy, eggs, legumes, and fats such as vegetable oils, nuts, avocados. Do not overdo the portions when you eat. Drink lots of water or unsweetened herbal teas.

It may take some time for your body to get used to this routine. It is necessary to be patient. During hunger attacks, it is suggested to drink a cup of unsweetened coffee or tea. Do workouts regularly and eat protein to avoid losing muscle mass. No matter when the training is placed during the day, the most hearty meal of the day should be after training. A lack of sleep could cause weight gain. Try to get enough sleep and rest.

Intermittent fasting is not for everyone, but it is a good method of reducing body fat. However, the diet must be kept under control by avoiding foods like hamburgers, pizzas and French fries. The goal remains to try to eat healthily and to follow a balanced diet.

Fasting and exercise

Food abstinence in combination with physical exercise leads to low insulin levels, a very important element for burning fat and preventing diabetes. Being over weighted can interfere with insulin's ability to lower sugar levels in blood. In addition, the body learns to process the food more efficiently in this time frame.

During fasting period, while training few things should be kept in mind. If the goal is to lose weight, it is important to reduce calories moderately, such losing the 0.5-1% of body fat. The ideal is, in routine training sessions, to increase proteins by 25%, such respecting the caloric intake and preserving lean muscle mass.

On the other side, those who wants to combine intense workouts and fasting should consult a doctor.

CONCLUSION

The intent of this book is to inform people conditioned by unrealistic weight loss diets imposed by fashions in advance. Even more ambitious is the idea that this work can educate the younger generations to live a correct dietary lifestyle, suitable for preventing obesity and all health risks deriving from incorrect nutrition.

Eating is one of the most important actions in our life that goes far beyond simple physiological satisfaction. How and what you eat depends both on the resources offered by the territory and on family habits and the relationship that is behind people and food. An old adage says: "you are what you eat, so don't be fast, cheap, easy or fake".

Traditional diets are based on decreasing calories, a very effective approach for those who want to lose excess weight. On the other hand, however, there is an increase in the desire for prohibited foods from a psychological point of view, with binge eating that risks frustrating the work done with the diet. To avoid this frustration, Sirt Diet intervenes to help, because it is based on the inclusion and not on the exclusion of food, without particular renunciations.

The Latin motto "menssana in corporesano" represents a valid expression of that healthy ambition that each individual should cultivate. The incorrect intake of food can be one of the main factors in the onset of diseases due to an excess of introduced calories, compared to those consumed. If sedentary lifestyles are added to this, the risk of incurring overweight and obesity becomes certainty. The low-calorie Sirt diet, is essentially based on a reasoned and varied combination of foods, and a diet aimed at achieving weight loss with the harmonious development of the organism.

For this reason it is necessary to replace a traditional low-calorie food program with all that sirt foods offer. The purpose of this diet is to accompany and support the individual during a not simple process of change, which involves the acquisition of a different dietary and physical lifestyle.

Avoiding many tasty foods is a bad habit, because the body is deprived of the necessary need for important nutrients. The lean genes responsible for repairing and rejuvenating cells accelerate their activity by drawing on fat reserves and increasing disease resistance. The same goal can be achieved without starving, by eating genetically rich Sirt foods, "sirtuins", considered to be super regulators of metabolism. They influence our ability to burn fat, the mechanisms that regulate longevity, mood and improve memory.

A complete approach to embarking on a new lifestyle is achieved when the diet is integrated with physical activity. Healthy eating behavior places the person's wellness philosophy at the center of attention, to foster a state of psycho-physical balance. Achieving a correct body weight must be achieved both by controlling nutrition and by making a more physically active life.

Only in this way it is possible to prevent obesity and other pathologies.

Considering that to this must be added environmental and genetic risk factors, the complexity of the elements involved, makes it clear that it is necessary to intervene, where possible, in an early manner.

In particular, as regards nutrition, prevention on eating must start from childhood and should become an heritage for the personal culture of every human being.

In many countries, with the aim of providing indications on how to eat, public institutions and scientific bodies have developed specific guidelines, aimed at defining and disseminating the basic information for a balanced diet aimed at well-being.